Harnessing the Wind

Chronic Fatigue Syndrome and My Son

by

Shanon McQuown

authorHOUSE™

1663 LIBERTY DRIVE, SUITE 200
BLOOMINGTON, INDIANA 47403
(800) 839-8640
WWW.AUTHORHOUSE.COM

First published by AuthorHouse 05/04/05

ISBN: 1-4184-7174-7 (e)
ISBN: 1-4184-3952-5 (sc)

Printed in the United States of America
Bloomington, Indiana

This book is printed on acid-free paper.

Do not let anyone treat you as if you're unimportant because you are young. Instead, be an example to the believers with your words, your actions, your love, your faith and your pure life. 1 Timothy 4:12

Table of Contents

Anthony:

Priceless One

Anthony, I am moved to tears every time I take a moment to think of what a gift God has given to me in you. You are
the best child I have ever known, and I can hardly believe I raised you. With all of the errors I've made in my past and all
of the things I don't know, you have always shown how proud you were of your mom and how sure you were that I would "kick
butt" for you.
You are, have always been and will always be a blessing to your mother. Watching you rise to face this battle has
made you into a hero in my eyes. I admire your strength and
determination. I'm proud of you! I look forward to seeing the man you're going to be. May the Lord keep you always
on the path of His choosing.

I love you so much. God loves you even more!

Mom: *Anthony, what would you say to other children who have CFIDS?*

Anthony: *I'd tell them to never give up.*

Gratitude

I have so many people to thank for standing beside us on this journey. My deepest thanks goes to my Heavenly Father for blessing me with such a wonderful son. I thank my mother for always being supportive and loving of us. I thank my father for editing this book and giving me a love for the written word.

I thank my friends on the CFS-P and Pediatric Network lists for their support, knowledge, encouragement and love. Fayth and Marissa, thank you for your unconditional love and support. Thank you Mary Z. Robinson for taking the time to encourage, educate and point me in the right directions. I'm indebted to Michelle Banks for her encouragement, friendship, love and educational information.

Thank you Bobbi S. for being the first mother of a boy with CFS to walk beside me. Becky, thank you for being there for me in the middle of the night when the journey was so new to us. Janet and Dani, Linda and Megan, Kim, Kaytlin and Clarence, I thank you for welcoming us into your homes and making us feel as if we were a part of your families.

Thank you Nicole, Amy and Samantha for telling me how it feels to be YPWCs (young people with CFS). Thank you Nicole and Amy for reaching out to Anthony on the Internet when CFS robbed him of his friends.

Thanks to Lynette Lewis, Mary-Beth Jones, Nicole Schwab and Maureen Winstead for supporting me as I tried to work and battle all comers for Anthony's health and education.

Pastor Dennis Rupert, you don't comprehend how important it was that you took the time to hang out with Anthony. Going to the movies and/or just spending time talking to him were equally important. He didn't get out much without your efforts. Thank you for being a strong and consistent male in Anthony's life.

Kristen, Amy and Karin, I thank you for letting Anthony live vicariously through your emails. You didn't give up when he didn't answer. You were true friends.

I extend my sincerest gratitude to Dr. Norman Bernstein for being the first to tie all of the symptoms together and give them a name. Dr. Barrington Bowser, words can't express
how grateful I am to you for stepping in with authority when we felt we had nowhere else to turn. Dr. Peter Rowe, I thank you for speaking to me after a conference three years ago and referring me to a great physical therapist in our area. Aaron Rathgeb (physical therapist extraordinaire), thank you, THANK YOU for helping my son regain so much of what he'd lost. Thank you also, Aaron, for the friendship you extended to Anthony.

Thank you to ALL of his teachers (Mr. Southwick, Dr. Gates, Mrs. Maddox, Mrs. Gooding, Mrs. Snively, Mrs. Mahew, Mr. Strackbein, Mr. Hodge, Mr. Ohmstead, Mrs.

Summerville, Mrs. Reed, Mrs. Danko, and Mrs. Dunn). Your flexibility, open-mindedness and creativity made it possible for Anthony to soar with the eagles.

Thank you to Anthony's case manager, Erin Welch, for being diligent, consistent, persistent, dependable and compassionate when managing Anthony's educational program. Thank you for relentlessly seeking ways to make things happen and always asking the question, "Why not?"

To the administrators, Mrs. Southerland and Mr. Stemple, thank you for sticking with us. Thanks for the progress we've made due to your open hearts and your willingness to keep fighting for Anthony's education.

Mrs. Platt, thank you for not turning your back on us when the battle placed us on opposite sides. Thank you for acknowledging the strengths and weaknesses on both sides of the fence and utilizing the strengths in all areas. We always knew and trusted you to be a fair and caring woman and time has proven it to be so. You are the example of what a special education supervisor should be. I praise you for the manner in which you endeavor to look out for the child's best interest. I pray that others will learn from you. My son has truly been blessed because of your efforts.

Debbie Fulz and Martha Myers, thank you for helping me increase my knowledge of the process of special-education service. Thank you for going with me to meetings and reining me in when I became to emotionally "heated." You helped me discover the best path for Anthony to have his rights and needs met.

To all of you, I express my love, my joy, my prayers and God's many blessings. You have all been an inspiration as I've watched you try to "Harness the Wind."

Forward

At the age of 14, my son, Anthony, was diagnosed with Chronic Fatigue Syndrome (CFS) also known as Chronic Fatigue and Immune Dysfunction Syndrome (CFIDS) on January 2, 2001. I spent the year prior to his diagnosis trying to figure out what had happened to change my son so drastically. Once his illness was diagnosed, the race was on to find physicians and therapists who were knowledgeable about the disease, and to find possible treatments. I hate to think of how many children and their parents are left in despair because doctors focus their efforts entirely toward depression while the physical symptoms are being ignored.

Anthony continually endured questions from medical professionals; "Are you depressed? Do you have thoughts of hurting yourself? Do you have thoughts of killing yourself? Do you have a plan (To kill yourself)?" When his body hurt, they assumed he was depressed. When he experienced digestive dysfunction, they assumed it was caused by depression. It seemed like we were in a never-ending and unproductive cycle. My son became frustrated with the questions. He could not figure out why — no matter what physical symptom for which he was being seen — it would be diagnosed as caused by depression.

We eventually felt insulted by the questions, but we are now able to look back and consider them almost comical. For depression to be secondary to a chronic illness is not uncommon. It is not surprising that, with the roller coaster of cognitive, immune, muscular and joint difficulties, depression might also come and go.

Does Anthony have a plan? Anthony and I have had several "plans" since he became ill; and when one plan proves to be unproductive, we recover and try another. Unfortunately, man has yet to develop a cure that works for everyone. Fortunately, our Heavenly Father does have a plan for us. *For I know the plans I have for you, plans to prosper you and not harm you, plans to give you hope and a future. Jeremiah 29:11*

Anthony's dream, since early childhood, has been to become a medical research scientist. Now he feels it is logical for him to be one who has CFS. He believes this journey will give him an increased understanding and compassion for others who suffer with the symptoms of recognized illnesses and illnesses that have yet to be given a name. I believe Anthony's illness serves as a motivation to find cures for others.

We are so fortunate that the Lord provided us with a wonderful team of physicians and a physical therapist who work well together on my son's behalf. It has been a long journey. It looks as if we still have farther to go. Yet, we are quite aware of the blessings we have received along the way.

Anthony and I have drawn closer to God and drawn strength from every adversity that has crossed our path. Emboldened, we now reach out to others. We don't claim to have all of the answers; we just know that we must continue fighting, not only for ourselves, but also for others who are feeling hopeless.

May this book bless you with hope, laughter and love. Know that our prayers go out to you wherever you are on your journey with CFS.

Rejoicing in Him Always!
Anthony's mom a.k.a. Shanon

Chapter One:
Introduction to a Warrior

Anthony was born at 12:36 a.m. on July 29, 1986. From the moment he was born, he became the biggest blessing I had ever experienced. He was adorable, and by all appearances, healthy.

He has been an extraordinary child from the moment he arrived. With his eyes, he tried to track my mother's voice in the delivery room. He has forever been curious about everything in his surroundings. I remember how I looked forward to him learning to roll over, until he tried to roll off the couch when he was only two weeks old. I looked forward to the day he could crawl…until I discovered crawling meant he would soon learn to climb. I could not blink my eyes and hope he'd be in the same position he'd been in just moments before. I yearned for the day he would walk, until I experienced the first of his many falls. I should be the skinniest woman on earth, because I have been running after Anthony ever since!

His mind was brilliant. He began reading books at the age of three. He always wanted to learn everything about everything. "Why?" quickly became his mantra. I think every mother tires of the "why" questions and the pretense that Mommy knows everything. He soon learned that he could find the answers to his questions for himself.

Anthony has always had a love of ALL animals, including dreaded insects that I had to force myself to tolerate. Before Anthony was born I had the rigid belief that anything that had more than four legs was to be kept a reasonable distance (maybe on Pluto) away from me. One day, maybe

I'll get my Academy Award for the skill I employed to mask the blanche I felt whenever he would want to examine or observe some "cute, little, furry," many-legged creature. As a toddler, Anthony startled me by screaming, as I was about to close a sliding door. I thought I had closed his little hand in the door, but to him, it was something much more serious. I had been insensitive enough to try to close the door while there was a helpless caterpillar trapped in the door's tracking. We had to find the perfect stick to pick up the perfect caterpillar to put on the underside of a perfect leaf so a hungry bird could not eat the perfect caterpillar. Then, and only then, could the world continue to rotate on its axis.

As he grew, he enjoyed playing several sports and musical instruments. He was popular, friendly, intelligent, compassionate and understanding. He usually tried to hide the telltale hint of a smirk that warned of a joke or trick he was plotting. His laughter filled my house and my heart.

Fortunately, we were blessed with a great relationship. I tell you this, because I want you to know the child I had before CFS reared its ugly head. I distinguish between then and now because the child I have now is not the same child I had before.

There were several stages leading to us coming to terms with CFS. I was, at first, unaware of what was happening, and unfortunately, I trusted his doctor who led me to the world of denial. The next stage was experiencing a deep, wrenching grief. At one stage, we were angry at the world. Finally, we have come to an acceptance. Acceptance does not mean giving up or being defeated. It simply means that I accept Anthony as he is today. I accept that he knows how he's feeling. I accept that sometimes,

it is necessary to learn new ways to help Anthony do the things he used to do with ease. I continue to have hopes and dreams for Anthony. I also encourage him to dream for

himself. I help him discover new avenues to reach each one of them.

Why are we not in a pit of pity? Why have we not given up? From where does our strength come? We have Jesus. He is our Light, our Provider, our Refuge, my husband and Anthony's father.

Anthony is not a victim. He is a warrior! Anthony's testimony is stronger because of the CFS in his life. Hanging on to faith is much easier when you travel on calm and crystal seas. We hang on to God when a crisis comes our way and repeatedly, He carries us through. Our moments of joy are fuller in the appreciation of the blessings and mercies he sends our way. *That is why, for Christ's sake, I delight in weakness, in insults, in hardships, in persecutions, in difficulties. For when I am weak, then I am strong. ~ 2 Corinthians 12:10*

Chapter Two:
The First Hint of Rough Waters

At the age of two, Anthony suffered a febrile seizure and was hospitalized. At the time, there was no definite explanation for it. Subsequently, we learned that any time Anthony's body tried to fight infection, his temperature would spike and bring on the dreaded seizures.

I can still feel the emotions of the day of the first seizure. I felt panic, fear and shock. I felt absolutely inadequate to help my child. I wanted to break down and cry, but I knew if I fell apart, the medical staff in the emergency room would have made me leave his side. As they performed a spinal tap, I tried to look as if I were stronger than I actually felt.

That night, beside his hospital bed, I recalled the words of a poem I learned when I was a teenager.

God's Lent Child

"I'll lend you for a little while, a child of mine," He said.
"For you to love while he lives and mourn when he is dead."
"It may be six or seven weeks, or thirty years or three."
"But will you, 'till I call him back, take care of him for me?"

"He'll bring his charm to gladden you and should his stay be brief,"
"You'll have his lovely memories as solace for your grief?"
"I cannot promise he will stay, since all from earth must

return,"
"But there are lessons taught down there I want this child
to learn."

"I looked the wide world over in my search for teachers
true,"
"And from the throngs that crowd life's way, I have
selected you."
"Now will you give him all your love, nor think the labor
in vain,"
"Nor hate Me when I come around to take him back
again?"

"I fancy that I hear you say, 'Dear Lord, Thy will be
done.'"
'For all the joy this child has brought, all fateful risks we
run.'
'We'll shelter him with tenderness, we'll love him while
we may,'
'And for the happiness we've known, we'll forever
grateful stay.'

But you came 'round to call for him much sooner than
we'd planned…
Dear Lord, forgive our grief and help us understand.
~Author Unknown

The words to the poem came to me so vividly that night,
I got on my knees at Anthony's bedside and cried out to
God for the first time in years. I told Him, "I know that
Anthony truly belongs to you, but know that I love him
too. Please don't take him from me now. He's all I have.

If you'll allow him to stay with me a little longer, I'll put him in a Christian school, and he'll grow up knowing and loving you."

In hindsight, it's funny that I didn't even think of dedicating my own life to Jesus at that moment. I just knew in my heart that I needed to do it for Anthony. I never forgot my vow and true to my word, when Anthony was old enough, I enrolled him in Christian preschool.

I had to help him learn memory verses from the Bible. Anthony ended up explaining the verses to me with that, "I know that I know, because God said so" faith of a child. I envied him, but I couldn't believe it could be that simple. We moved to Northern Virginia and I immediately enrolled him in a Christian kindergarten. Within two weeks of the move, we met Tony and Cindy, the parents of Anthony's favorite classmate, Ashley. By the following weekend, we had been welcomed into Tony and Cindy's church family and I formed my own personal relationship with Jesus.

Anthony's life was filled with love, laughs and activity. His antics provided me with endless hours of hidden laughter. Everything in his world was climbed on, jumped on or jumped from. He was bright, handsome, polite and humble. When he was five, he was told he was cute. My "humble" child responded, "I know, because God put many blessings in my cup!"

Anthony's health continued to trouble him. He repeatedly had leg aches. However, physicians quickly labeled them "growing pains." Eventually, Anthony was sent to a children's hospital where a pediatric rheumatologist gave a diagnosis of hyper mobility syndrome (double-jointed). Resulting "loose joints" caused Anthony to hyperextend his knees on a regular basis, only to be left with severe aches that lasted for days.

Anthony also had asthma and frequent nosebleeds. He frequently pulled muscles and ligaments in his legs, and I marveled at his ability to still walk into the hospital on his own. This is what made me realize that Anthony had inherited a high pain threshold from my father and me. Looking back, it makes sense. Anthony has dealt with some degree of pain most of his life. As children will do, Anthony managed to adapt to his circumstances and led an active life of baseball, soccer, basketball, bicycling, roller blading and Tae Kwon Do.

Additionally, it seemed as though Anthony suffered disproportionately from contracting colds and viruses. For example, if someone had a cold, he'd end up with bronchitis. If someone else had the sniffles, Anthony would end up with a sinus infection. He even managed to contract Scarlet Fever! Nobody we knew had it. More than 10 years have passed, and I'm still trying to figure out where it came from! Nonetheless, despite the frequent medical problems, Anthony was full of joy, energy and love. He was happiest child I knew.

Chapter Three Year One:
Mutiny of Anthony's Body

In the sixth grade, Anthony had a bout of problems with his digestive system and tore his ACL ligament. He also continued to suffer with his asthma and opportunistic colds and infections. Subsequently, he missed a lot of school. His grades started dropping, mainly because he kept forgetting to turn in assignments that I had watched him complete. Teachers reported that he would even forget to turn in work that they had done together as a class. They told me they felt he wasn't paying attention, because he would frequently lay his head on his desk. I decided to hold Anthony back a year and let him try again at a new school. I knew something wasn't right, but I couldn't put my finger on it. Hindsight is wonderful. I wish I knew then what I know now.

At the new school, Anthony never seemed to get it together. He had many friends who graced my home with "teenage-boy noise." He played in the school band. He just couldn't seem to hold it together with his grades. My worst goof in motherhood came at this point. Doctors were telling me that nothing was wrong with Anthony. Some teachers professed that he just wasn't "living up to his potential."

I took Anthony on a ride one evening with the intention of trying to help him realize what he was throwing away by not applying himself. I reminded Anthony of how brilliant his brain was and told him that Martin Luther King and others involved in the Civil Rights Movement died so that he could have the opportunity to put his brain to good use. I admonished him by saying that it's like spitting on their graves when he didn't apply his best effort.

Anthony reflected on what I said and tried desperately to reach his former academic levels, but now, I know he couldn't. Anthony was having cognitive problems that he didn't understand or have a clue how to explain to me. Consequently, he never told me.

In the seventh grade, Anthony's digestive tract suffered severe motility (movement) dysfunction. To be honest, I can't adequately describe what he went through. I have struggled with how much to publish about this time period. After many days of indecisiveness, I sought Anthony's input and permission. He insisted that I tell it all with the hope of possibly sparing another child the agony that he endured. What follows is quite graphic.

In the late fall of 1999, I noticed that Anthony, at some times, walked with an odd gait: his shoulders hunched forward and he walked slowly. When I asked

Anthony about it, he responded with complaints of severe leg pain. I took him to see his rheumatologist who prescribed an anti-inflammatory. I asked for further testing to identify the cause of the pain. This was a long, tedious endeavor that never resulted in a positive diagnosis or solution. I also noticed that he spent more and more time in bed. I assumed it was because he was a teenager and needed more rest. Even when he was awake, he was on the bed reading books or playing video games. Additionally, he wasn't hanging out with his friends as much as he used to. At the time, I was attending night classes at a local college, so I didn't really get to see the full picture until Christmas vacation.

One evening as I sat in the living room, I noticed Anthony slowly making his way down the hall. I asked him if his legs were the only source of his pain. He replied that his stomach felt queasy and was hurting. I asked him when he had last moved his bowels. He told me it had been a few days. I had him lift his shirt so I could feel his stomach. His belly was rock hard. I thought that he might have been constipated, and with little success, attempted to address the problem with over-the-counter stool softeners and laxatives.

Subsequently, Anthony's doctor tried various remedies including a high-fiber diet and medications. With each attempt to move his bowels, only partial voiding was achieved. Eventually, Anthony stopped eating and began experiencing what he called "sulfur burps." He told me those burps tasted awful. I can assure you that they smelled even worse! Anthony's appetite was almost non-existent. I cannot remember a sadder Christmas in Anthony's life. In the past, Anthony would frequently come into the kitchen as I prepared the holiday meal, to taste whatever he could sneak or beg. He would then enthusiastically devour his favorite Christmas foods. He would have seconds and, after playing outside for awhile, he would have thirds and fourths. The Christmas of 1999, Anthony sat at the table looking longingly at the food, taking a few bites before asking if he could be excuse from the table.

The muscles in his legs began to atrophy from lack of use. He became exceptionally weak. In his worst moments, he would crawl wherever he needed to go in the house. Still, nobody could tell me what was wrong with my son. He began spending the majority of the day in bed.

When the medications the doctors prescribed attempted to work, Anthony passed "stones" that were about the diameter of a tennis ball and as hard as rocks – parts of a solid mass that had formed inside his body. When he'd go into the restroom, he'd scream in pain. Eventually, these stones caused the skin to split on their way out. This resulted in inflammation and infection. The doctor recommended long soaks in the tub. Anthony would scream in pain as the water made contact with the splits. He'd beg for me not to make him get into the tub and plead for me to let him get out. The ointment the doctor prescribed was not successful in healing the torn places. Tears still fill my eyes when I think about it for more than a brief moment. We sought help from family physicians and emergency room staff. They all seemed to have faith in whatever treatment they tried. My faith in their faith was not so secure.

During this period, Anthony time out of bed was almost non-existent. He slept the majority of the day and was unable to eat much of anything. Sometimes he was absolutely out of his mind in pain. Other times, he was completely exhausted.

Michael Joe, Anthony's friend since birth, was the only friend who asked to come to visit, because he was worried about Anthony. The last time he came, he sat in

15

Anthony's room while Anthony slept. He just wanted to be near Anthony. When I'd go to check on them, the look on Michael Joe's face broke my heart. His courage and determination to stand by his friend inspired me. During the moments when Anthony would awaken, Michael Joe made a great effort to speak with Anthony as if nothing was wrong. Michael Joe only recently expressed to me how afraid he was for Anthony. Anthony doesn't remember much of those visits, but I'll never forget the friend who stuck with Anthony when it looked like Anthony would die.

As time passed, I became more and more concerned. I was sure there was a blockage. I worried that he'd end up needing a colostomy if something wasn't done soon. Toward the end of the crisis, Anthony regurgitated something that looked like and had the odor of something that one should only find in a toilet. I knew enough about human anatomy to know that if Anthony's system was blocked, some of the toxins could leak through the lining of his intestines into the rest of his body. I prayed for God to send someone to help because I couldn't get anyone to listen to me.

Finally, Anthony was referred to a pediatric gastroenterologist (stomach doctor). This time, I was prepared. As morbid as it may sound, I froze one of the "stones" to show the doctor what was coming out of Anthony. Dr. Graham examined Anthony and quickly realized that there was a problem. He prescribed a strong medication that he'd hoped would solve the problem. When the medication proved unsuccessful, Anthony was hospitalized. At this point, Anthony was about 5'4" and weighed approximately 90lbs soaking wet.

When Anthony was admitted into the hospital, he was terrified to hear the doctor describe the procedure that was to be implemented. When the time came for Anthony's IV to be inserted, he was blessed with two "Pet Visitor" golden retrievers. The male nuzzled Anthony in sympathy as the enema was administered. God knew that Anthony's love of animals surpassed his fear of the needles and the enema. God also knew exactly what Anthony needed at that moment and provided it in abundance. *And my God shall supply all your needs according to His riches and glory. ~ Philippians 4:19*

An NG (nose to stomach) tube had to be inserted to attack the blockage from the top of Anthony's body. This was one of the few, if not the only, time that I truly hated being a mother. For some reason, the nurse had difficulty getting the NG tube inserted in the correct position. As the nurse withdrew the uncooperative tube, Anthony gagged and sputtered. Nothing I did was adequate to comfort my son. He cried and I held it in. My heart ached so terribly for Anthony. Finally, on the third attempt, the tube was correctly placed. He still looks back on that episode as the worst part of being in the hospital. I stayed at his bedside and prayed all night for the treatment to work.

I also had time to reflect on my relationship with Anthony. I thought about how Anthony longed for braids and how I had refused to allow him to grow his hair. It was so obvious that the dreaded braids were nothing in comparison to not

17

having my son with me anymore. Alone, in the darkness, at my son's hospital bedside, I again cried out desperately to God. "I know that Anthony's still yours. I know he belongs to you. Again, I am begging you to allow him to stay with me a while longer. To show that I have dedicated him to you, I will learn to braid his hair and I will never cut his hair again."

Anthony was unconscious for the next day. He remembers nothing. Fortunately, the dual administration of the medication successfully disintegrated the blockage that night. I would never have imagined being so elated to see such a horrid mess! I cried. I rejoiced. I thanked God for giving Dr. Graham the knowledge and the determination to relieve my son's discomfort.

Dr. Graham followed Anthony's case for another full year. He prescribed treatment to help Anthony's intestines shrink back to normal size and learn to function properly on their own again. Anthony HATED taking the medicine. At times, I had to chase him around to make him take it. Once, I even pinned him down until he relented. It probably would have been comical to someone observing us, but that was serious business.

It was a long road. Anthony still wrinkles his nose at the thought of those medications. He never wants to even look at them again. I pray that there will never again be the need for Anthony to take those medications.

I have not cut Anthony's hair again since the hospitalization. His hair is now longer than mine. Anthony's long braids are my Ebenezer, my reminder of all that God has carried us through. Any time I feel frustrated with Anthony, the hair reminds me of what is important and what I almost lost.

Some might wonder why I included this segment...It draws attention to a child's simple logic. Anthony later told me that he "knew" he was dying. He didn't think anything could be done to help him. He said he hurt so badly that he "wanted" to die. I told him he should NEVER hide anything like that again. He was fighting the battle, attempting to face it courageously (in his own way) and losing terribly. I assured him that if something could be done, I'd always find a way. Teenagers are in the weird position of feeling like they're grown-up without having the reasoning skills or the life experiences of adults. We must remember that they're not little grown-ups, no matter how tall they are. We can't assume they will tell us everything. We must remember to ask.

Since writing this segment, Anthony's past suffering has helped to spare other children from suffering the same fate or worse. Parents have called me, because their children's symptoms reminded them of something they heard me say. Some have been close to the point at which Anthony was hospitalized. Anthony begins to pray for these children as soon as I tell him about them. Then, he smiles a glorious smile when they have a happier outcome than his. He knows that his suffering was NOT in vain.

Chapter Four Year Two:
The "C" Monster Raises Its Ugly Head

Anthony's physical symptoms gradually improved. With physical therapy, he temporarily regained some of his strength. He still did not return to his normal energy levels. He easily became disoriented. Once, he was three hours late coming home because he got lost in the neighborhood we had lived in for three years. He was panicked and in the midst of an asthma attack when he finally made it home. It was odd, but the asthma attack took priority over the disorientation. At the time, we couldn't imagine what was happening to Anthony's cognitive ability.

That summer, we tried to visit the local amusement park. We purchased season tickets on a yearly basis. On the first, and only, visit that year, Anthony was only able to walk halfway into the park. He was overcome by pain and weakness in his legs. He was so exhausted that he had to be carried out piggyback. Anthony has not been back to the park again. It grieves me because he used to enjoy the park to the fullest. Now, he can't walk the distance, withstand the sensory overload or tolerate being banged around on rides. He quietly accepted the circumstances.

One of the joys of visiting the park was sharing the many smells, joyous sounds and sights of the people and attractions. With sensory overload, too many lights, noises, movements and smells overwhelm Anthony's ability to process them. His energy levels rapidly crash, and he puts his head down and closes his eyes. He uses his head phones to drown out outside noises. To the person who doesn't know, it seems like Anthony is withdrawing. In actuality, it is a comfort measure.

Anthony began complaining of other symptoms (chest pain, sore throat, muscle and joint pain, headaches and extreme fatigue). He usually became confused and frustrated when trying to explain his symptoms to his doctor. One day after the doctor left the examining room, Anthony said to me, "I wish I could go to sleep and never wake up again." I realized my son was full of despair. When the doctor returned, I told him what Anthony said, and we agreed to get Anthony in to see a counselor.

The counselor was helpful assisting Anthony in facing his fears of medical treatment. Once his digestive condition improved, so did his demeanor. I was pleased with the progress he was making coping with being ill and all the subsequent testing he had to endure.

When the new school year rolled around, Anthony attempted to make it to school again. His grades were marvelous. I was truly hopeful. He was, however, too exhausted to make it to school, although he slept anywhere from 13 to 22 hours a day.

Finally, his teachers, school nurse and school counselor became concerned about the things they were observing at school. It took extraordinary amounts of time for him to travel between classes. Once he arrived, he was exhausted and would promptly collapse with his head down on his desk. Again, he began to forget to turn in homework and class work. The school nurse would send him home because of low-grade fevers and swollen lymph nodes. I was relieved that someone else was seeing that something

23

was wrong. I was truly at my wit's end. Anthony, at this point, was 5'6" and weighed only about 104 lbs.

When the school started sending him home, repeatedly, I took Anthony to Dr. P. (the new general practitioner.) *Anthony's pediatrician had moved out of state.* Mercilessly, Dr. P. would berate me for not "making" Anthony go to school. He told me that Anthony "looked fine" to him. Dr. P. was a runner. I suppose the rail of a child that Anthony had become **would** look "fine" to him. I'd restated the purpose for our visit. We argued about our difference of opinion. I tried to explain that he didn't know Anthony. I tried to tell him of the child I knew before Anthony became ill. Again, he told me nothing was wrong with Anthony, and I just needed to **make** him go to school. I became so angry that tears filled my eyes. Anthony said, "Come on, Mom. Let's go. I'm fine." I still get angry when I think about this, because Anthony was trying to protect me. I pleaded with God to allow me to "lay hands" on this man. God restrained me because He knew it wouldn't have been for the purpose of healing. Instead, I told Dr. P. I did *make* Anthony go to school and one hour later, the school would call me *making* me come back and pick him up. In what I saw as an attempt at intimidation, Dr. P. announced, "Well, maybe I just need to talk to the school." I gladly handed him the phone number.

I was told that when he called, he made it obvious that he thought I was overreacting. I was blessed that the person he spoke to had the fortitude to give the response, "Well, let *me* tell *you* what *we've* observed here at the school." Then, she explained the difficulty they had watched Anthony having. I was fortunate that she had known Anthony before he became incapacitated and could see for herself his drastic decline.

Dr. P. never called me after speaking to the person at the school. The next week, after being summoned once again to pick Anthony up from school, we entered Dr. P's office full of trepidation, but wanting so desperately to have some hope. He sneered, "I don't know what *devastating* disease you think your son has, but he's fine." I told him that I hoped my son didn't have a "devastating illness," but I hoped he could tell me what was wrong. By this time, I had become firmly convinced that this man was the spawn of Satan! How could someone drip so freely with acidic sarcasm and swear an oath to help people, not do them physical or psychological harm? Dr. P. casually mentioned that Anthony's latest blood-test results revealed that Anthony had elevated levels of Epstein Barr Virus/EBV (virus that causes mono). When asked what that meant and if that could have been causing Anthony's symptoms, he informed me that there was no way to know when Anthony had been infected or how long the levels would remain elevated.

I, then, asked the Dr. P. what he knew about CFS. He told me he'd never heard of a boy Anthony's age having it. I just looked at him. I guess it wasn't just a look. Anthony actually calls it *"the look."* It's the look we mothers give our children when they're one step from big trouble. Anthony swears it will melt the skin off a person's face and make him go blind if he is not wearing sunglasses.

Not to be shaken by "the look," Dr. P. said, in a condescending tone, "If it will make you feel better, I'll give him a referral to see an Infectious Disease Specialist." I replied, "It would make me feel better if *somebody* was doing *anything* for my child."

As we left the office, that day, we were given a referral to see Dr. Bernstein. We felt a glimmer of hope. To Anthony, he was being sent to yet another doctor to poke and prod his body and then tell him nothing was wrong. How do you keep a child from becoming discouraged when those he looks to for help only ignore his desperate need?

When we got home from Dr. P's office, I talked to Anthony and said something like, "Anthony, you've got to learn to be an advocate for yourself. I can't remember all of your symptoms, and you forget by the time we get in the doctors' offices. We need to make a list of the things that bother you." That evening, we made a list from head to toe (internal and external). I tried to maintain my composure, as the list took on a life of its own. When we were finally finished, I asked Anthony why he didn't tell me all of his symptoms before then. He explained that he didn't know they weren't normal since some of the symptoms had been with him as long as he could remember. I felt a lump rise in my throat as we addressed his pains. I was shocked to learn that his skin even hurt him sometimes. He confessed that it sometimes hurt him to be hugged.

Some of the symptoms Anthony was coping with at that time were:

- Fatigue/exhaustion
- Insomnia, Hypersomolence, or sleep pattern reversal
- Muscle pains (all over the body)
- Joint pains (wrist, elbows, fingers, hips, knees, ankles, toes and jaw)
- Headaches
- Heat/Cold Sensitivities
- Skin stinging, burning or sensitive to the touch (all over)
- Sharp chest, neck, back and side pains
- Muscle spasms (legs, arms, hands and fingers will jump or twitch unexpectedly)
- Frequent upper-respiratory infections
- Dizziness, nausea, weakness, loss of balance
- Tinnitis (ringing in ears)
- Sensitivities (light, odors, movement, noise)
- Cognitive difficulties (short-term memory lapses, multi-tasking difficulty, computation deficits, word-finding deficits, delayed response and processing time, shortened attention span, disorientation, dysgraphia)
- Vision (blurring, words "moving" on the page, eye pain)
  - *The more he was fatigued, the more his symptoms magnified.*
  - *The symptoms fluctuate throughout the day.*

We met with Dr. Bernstein. After he reviewed Anthony's symptom list and took his medical history, I braced for more ridicule. Anthony withdrew into himself as experience had taught him to do. Instead, Dr. Bernstein asked Anthony very specific questions in relation to each symptom. I watched Anthony peek over the wall of protection he had placed around himself. Was someone REALLY listening? After a long interview and exam, Dr. Bernstein told us that it sounded like Chronic Fatigue Syndrome, but he wanted to run more tests to rule out other disorders. Anthony wanted no more to do with blood work, but relented because he had hope that this time we would be given some answers. Finally, Anthony received a diagnosis. The monster had a name. We thought the battle would soon be over. In a perfect world, it would have been. Unfortunately, we do not live in a perfect world. The storm had just begun.

Chapter Five:
An Armada of Physicians

I feel it is imperative to share our experience with the seemingly endless list of doctors, because many CFS sufferers visit many doctors, seeking treatment, cures and hope for their vast assortment of symptoms.

Anthony was taken to many doctors in the search for the cause of all of his symptoms. He came to detest even the thought of walking into yet another doctor's office.

I am grateful that the Lord provided wise doctors who were able to break through the wall of protection Anthony had so skillfully begun to build up. I am also thankful for the ones who had the determination and the tenacity to keep looking for a cause. They ruled diseases out, while never appearing to blame Anthony for becoming sick.

I include this "Armada" because some important things were discovered in the midst of the confusion. I include it as an encouragement to those who suffer with this disease and question their need to follow through. YOU MUST RULE OUT OTHER DISEASES AND DISORDERS! Just because your child has been diagnosed with CFS doesn't mean nothing else could be going wrong in his body.

Whenever Anthony would first enter the office of a new physician, he said, he felt as if he'd been drawn into a typhoon. There are so many symptoms for the physician to investigate and so many symptoms for Anthony to remember. The physician and the Anthony could both be (understandably) overwhelmed. For the physicians who chose to ride out the storm and provide a "life jacket" for added safety, I applaud you for the effort and courage you've shown by not jumping ship as so many others have done in the past and might do in the future.

I offer this as encouragement to people with CFS. There ARE doctors out there who are willing to continue looking for the elusive cause. Dr. Graham was determined to figure out what had caused Anthony's digestive system to shut down so completely. He was the first physician who insisted on digging deeper to learn the identity of the culprit. He gave referrals to other specialists whose data allowed a diagnosis to be found.

Year One

Pediatrician:

Anthony was a patient of this doctor prior to his digestive dysfunction. He was seen mostly for meniscus injuries, asthma attacks, joint hyper-mobility, swollen and painful lymph nodes and upper respiratory infections. Sometimes Anthony had to wear braces on his legs to keep his knees from over-extending. When Anthony's digestive system started to malfunction, the doctor tried to remedy the problem. After the doctor had utilized all of the options at her disposal, she referred Anthony to a pediatric gastroenterologist. In the midst of the storm, the pediatrician moved and Anthony's insurer changed. We were forced to find another doctor.

Rheumatologist:

Anthony routinely saw a rheumatologist, Dr. K. At the beginning, Anthony was screened for Lupus to see if he had inherited the disease from me. He was given an anti-inflammatory to help with the pain in his legs. It didn't change Anthony's symptoms. This doctor went no further in searching for a diagnosis. In fact, after looking over my copy of Anthony's records, I discovered he wasn't taking it very seriously. In hindsight, I am a bit frustrated that the possibility of fibromyalgia was never even approached. Anthony had many of the symptoms. I often wonder if Anthony's condition would have deteriorated to the point at which it plunged had the rheumatologist looked deeper. I also found that the rheumatologist noted in his records, "It is possible he has a type of Marfan's syndrome." Remarkably, the first I knew of his suspicion was when I asked and paid for copies of all of Anthony's records a year later. In the notes and reports, I found a year's worth of noted pain complaints along with the glaring presence of the word "fatigue" repeatedly stated. Ironically, this doctor now professes to specialize in the treatment of Fibromyalgia.

Counselor:

When Anthony's digestive problems were almost at their peak and he had just about given up, I began to take him to a counselor. The counselor, Ms. M., was wonderful in helping Anthony deal with his hatred of needles and frustration of going from doctor to doctor. She taught him some relaxation techniques, and his anxiety over doctor visits and test decreased.

Almost a year later, once Anthony was diagnosed with CFS, her attitude toward both of us changed drastically. As most CFS sufferers and their caregivers have experienced, once you tell someone of a CFS diagnosis, they know the perfect cure that worked for someone they know. Ms. M. was no exception. She printed off some nutritional information for us. She also strongly recommended (or insisted) that Anthony begin Cranio Sacral Therapy with someone she knew. Anthony's insurance didn't cover this type of therapy. Her disappointment that we would not be going was made obvious.

Ms. M. set goals for Anthony that were focused on things that his body, at that time, was not capable of accomplishing. Appointments were scheduled at times when Anthony would normally be resting. Anthony was also on medications that made him groggy. Needless to say, his tired mind could not rise to the challenge cognitively. Anthony's responses to the counselor were short and most times monosyllabic. He realized she did not believe in CFS and withdrew from her. The harder she pushed, the further Anthony withdrew.

In the second year of counseling, my husband abandoned us. At this point, the counselor decided that Anthony's problem was depression and tried to get him to sign some paper in relation to hospitalization. My mother, who had taken him to the appointment, was never allowed to see the paper. When the psychiatrist entered the room, he stated that hospitalization "wasn't necessary" and did not sign off on it. Ms. M. sent a note home with my mother that said, "Shanon, I'd like to meet w/ the entire family the next session. (That's right! You, both grandparents and Anthony) I need all of your expert wisdom in helping Anthony through this problem. Please make at least five appointments where all can attend." I was shocked because Anthony had been diagnosed with CFS (a medical illness) long before my husband left. What had happened? Anthony said he didn't know what she was talking about. Mentally, I ran down a list of warning signs and couldn't imagine what she was alluding to. Anthony had been socializing more, during this period, than he had in the previous two years. His level of energy allowed for a little up time, and we had been excited about it. He was eating well and gaining weight. We both had to adjust to having to move in with my parents, and we were coping. We leaned on each other.

At the first family session, Ms. M. finally mentioned that Anthony was not willing to set goals or try to meet the ones she set for him. She felt he needed to make an effort or be hospitalized. We asked questions to try to have some clarity of her drastic suggestion and could not get any definitive answers. I watched Anthony during the entire meeting. There was an invisible cocoon around him.

I asked for and scheduled a private meeting with Ms. M. I asked her, if she truly felt that Anthony was so depressed that hospitalization was needed, why she didn't inform me. She again lamented over the fact that Anthony wasn't willing to set goals. She felt that he was isolated and depressed. (Depression had no longer been a major issue for Anthony once he knew he had a recognized illness.) She complained that he was isolated now that we had to move. I told her that Anthony was more active than he had been in two years and gave her examples. When she responded that she didn't know, I told her that she didn't ask Anthony or me. I told her that her focus was on the goals that she wanted Anthony to achieve. I informed her that Anthony was physically incapable of achieving those goals…thus rendering them invalid. I also addressed the fact that nobody, other than me, had the right to authorize Anthony to sign any papers. She told me that she felt threatened. (Where did this turn into *anything* about *her*?) I stayed on topic and stated that if she felt my son was suicidal or suffered from a major depressive disorder, it was her responsibility to inform me. Her response was, "Not necessarily." I reminded her that my son was only 14 years old and had no legal right to sign off on anything. She admitted that she didn't feel as if Anthony was suicidal. I was perplexed as I listened to her explain that the reason she was concerned was because Anthony was not having success setting physical goals. She was also concerned because Anthony had "stopped speaking to her." This is when a light bulb flashed somewhere in my mind. Her last statement kept replaying in my mind. Finally, I told her that the bottom line is that Anthony is no longer communicating with her. I told her that this was a waste of her time and Anthony's. I told her that Anthony would not be coming back.

I wondered why the goals *she* wanted to set for Anthony were so drastic instead of gradual steps. I wondered why everything depended on Anthony embracing *her* goals. My question was answered while I was going through Anthony's file at school and found a letter (parts of which were erroneous) that Ms. M had sent to Anthony's school six month's prior to wanting to hospitalize Anthony.

June 4, 2001

Dear xxxxxxx:

This letter is in response to our phone conversation this morning regarding my client Anthony xxxxx. This child has attended a total of 17 individual and family sessions with me beginning April 21, 2000 until the present. Initially, the family was concerned that Anthony might be depressed as a result of several issues: a previous acute medical condition which appeared to be life threatening and required hospitalization; continual physical pain and chronic exhaustion which was difficult to treat; his mother's chronic illness; and the on-going tension in the home around the past abuse of two half-brothers. The family has explored numerous physicians, specialists and diagnostic evaluations seeking help for Anthony. In the meantime, he has been diagnosed with Chronic fatigue Syndrome, Mononucleosis, some joint atrophy, which was alleviated with physical therapy; and Poland's Syndrome. Our staff Psychiatrist, Dr. R. has met with Anthony five times beginning December 19, 2000 until the present and prescribed Remeron for the depression.

According to Anthony, his physical symptoms have lessened, with the exception of chronic fatigue, pain in the tissues and occasional difficulty sleeping at night. With extended physical illness, which has been difficult to diagnose and treat, it is not unusual for one to experience feelings of depression, which add to the complexity of the situation. Presently, it appears that Anthony continues to have great difficulty maintaining stamina necessary to complete schoolwork in the home. The family reports that it has been very challenging for him to have a social life or pursue outside interests because of the continued physical symptoms. Anthony is making progress towards realizing a "normalized" lifestyle for a teen. Although difficult to predict, it would seem that Anthony in the coming year could regain capability to return to school with measured educational assistance for his difficulties."

I hope this letter is helpful. If you have further questions, call me at xxx xxxx.

Sincerely,
Ms. M

Family and Child Therapist

The first week of December 2000, Anthony had his first visit with the infectious disease specialist. The next week, full of hope for a diagnosis, we told Ms. M. of the doctor's suspicion that CFS might be the cause of Anthony's symptoms. She scheduled us for our first appointment with Dr. R., the psychiatrist, a little more than two weeks later. (Note: Anthony had been receiving therapy from Ms. M. for eight months before she suddenly decided to pull Dr. R. in on Anthony's case)

She is correct when she mentions the concern of depression over Anthony's health issues, but when she mentions family issues, she's way off the mark, because those events occurred in 1994. My "chronic illness" is named Lupus, and I was diagnosed in early 1990's.

After mentioning the numerous physicians, specialists and diagnostic evaluations, she states that Anthony has "in the meantime been diagnosed with CFS." (as if that's just a label to give it until they find out what's *really* wrong) Anthony has never been diagnosed with mono.

Dr. R was treating with low dosages of anti-depressants at levels appropriate for assistance with sleeping, not for depression. (See the section on Psychiatrist in reference to Dr. R's treatment protocol for Anthony.)

Anthony's only physical symptom that had lessened was of digestive origin. Chronic fatigue, pain and sleep difficulty are all classic symptoms of CFS. His stamina and difficulty with his social life are results of CFS. I don't know what kind of "normalized lifestyle for a teen" she thought Anthony was making progress towards. Our desire was to help Anthony discover what a normal lifestyle was for Anthony!

The last sentence (about Anthony regaining capability to return to school, with measured educational assistance for his difficulties) told me all I needed to know. This woman truly had no clue what she was dealing with in CFS. CFS is a monster, and it is real! She had also made a prediction that Anthony, to this day, is not able to "realize." Ms. M's opinion of Anthony's illness was based on assumptions. She secretively used her professional status try to foist her opinions on the school system. Time has proven her **wrong**. *For there is nothing hidden that will not be disclosed, and nothing concealed that will not be known or brought out into the open.~ Luke 8:17*

This therapist could have made such a positive impact in Anthony's life had she focused on helping Anthony learn to live WITH his CFS. Depression, secondary to *any* chronic illness, is NOT uncommon. Secondary or situational depression cannot be treated the same as major depressive disorder. Anthony felt as if he was getting blamed for becoming sick.

Psychiatrist:

Dr. R. had a quiet and serious affect. His nurse was intelligent and cheerful. The nurse joked around with Anthony as she took Anthony's intake information. The doctor took the time to explain anything he was doing. He answered Anthony's questions. In between sessions, I'm convinced that Anthony schemed to come up with the perfect question that would stump the doctor and his nurse.

Dr. R. was a blessing to the newly diagnosed Anthony. An anti-depressant was prescribed to take the edge off of the depression and help Anthony sleep. Dr. R. explained to us that he was giving Anthony a very low dosage. We were informed of the highest dosage Anthony could take before it would stop being therapeutic for his appetite and sleep. We were fortunate to find a psychiatrist who was familiar with the fact that many CFS patients have sensitivity to medications. Even a small dosage sometimes made Anthony almost too groggy to function.

Dr. R. wanted to keep Anthony's emotions on an even level. Dr. R. was also wise enough to recognize the difference in CFS symptoms and a Major Depressive Disorder.

Year Two

Pediatric Gastroenterologist:

Dr. Graham treated Anthony's digestive disruption during this period and was instrumental in getting physicians to keep looking. He recommended a treatment plan to help Anthony's digestive system return to normal function.

When Dr. Graham released Anthony from the hospital, Anthony weighed he weighed about 90 pounds. Dr. Graham continued to follow Anthony's case for the next year. He monitored Anthony's weight, appetite and motility.

Anthony's digestive system slowly returned to almost normal functioning. We still have to be careful about what he eats and how often his bowels move. We have not had another experience like the crisis we faced in the beginning of our journey.

Geneticist:

The first time we went to the geneticist, they ruled out Ehler Danlos Syndrome. It was noted that Anthony's joints were hyper-mobile. Nothing else was done.

A little more than a year later, after the infectious disease specialist found abnormalities in MRIs, we were referred back to the geneticist. An MRI revealed that Anthony was missing an left upper-chest muscle so completely that the specialist questioned if it had been surgically removed. He also has a smaller chest cavity and less lung capacity on the same side. He has a slight amount of webbing between his fingers.

This time, with specifics from the MRI and suspicions from the doctor, the geneticist noted that Anthony had Poland's Syndrome. Poland's Syndrome is another little-known congenital condition that consists of absence of chest muscle, absence of fingers, webbing between fingers, and/or reduced development of limbs.

Anthony's case is much-more mild than others I know with Poland's. What I wonder is, how did the same geneticist miss all of this the first time?

Physical Therapist One:

The muscles in Anthony's legs atrophied during the trial with his digestive system. Anthony was referred to physical therapy. His therapists were able to help Anthony regain some of the strength in his legs. His stamina was still not back to normal, but he was better that before. When Anthony's overall health crashed, Anthony could not return to this office, because it was not a provider accepted by his new insurance.

Orthopedist:

Anthony was referred to Dr. Sharps, the orthopedist. Dr. Sharps assessed and treated Anthony for his difficulties with mobility after his release from the hospital. Dr. Sharps was a cheerful man with a pleasant disposition. He joked with Anthony as he tried to discover how severe Anthony's deficiencies had become. Anthony tried to tell Dr. Sharps that he was fine. Dr. Sharps asked Anthony to squat down and then, with his arms straight out in front of him, stand up. Anthony attempted to stand up as if this task was simple… and then promptly fell over to the side. *This was the first doctor to look past Anthony's state of denial and show Anthony that his body was not at a condition of normal functioning. Dr. Sharps was kind and understanding. He was NEVER condescending.

Otolayrngologist:

A visit to the ear specialist led to a diagnosis of a mild hearing loss in Anthony's left ear and tinnitis. Anthony has experienced ringing in his ears (actually a high-pitched

squeal) since he was in elementary school. He thought it was normal. His hearing loss is funny because I remember how many headphones we replaced because he said *they* didn't "work right." We now know that it wasn't the headphones!

Cardiologist:

After an abnormal EKG on Anthony's heart, he was referred to a wonderful pediatric cardiologist, Dr. Moscowitz (name printed with permission). An echocardiogram revealed that Anthony had a mass in one of the ventricles of his heart. Anthony affectionately named this growth, "Bob." I was terrified.

Anthony's sense of humor kept me going. He joked, "Bob is so pushy. He came to visit without even asking for an invitation." The mass, Bob, was watched closely for changes. It was finally decided that Bob was probably a myocarditis scar left over from a virus. Hah! What virus?

When did Anthony have it? How did we miss it? Nobody had that answer.

The doctor also noted a mild thickening of the aortic and mitral valve. We then had to add another thing to the list of things we needed to watch closely.

Six months later, at the follow-up appointment, we were happy to learn that "Bob" hadn't changed in shape or size. Anthony was discharged from care, but told to return when Anthony turned 18.

*UPDATE: At the last mentioned appointment, Dr. Moscowitz cheerfully announced that it looked as if "Bob" had almost disappeared. He agreed that the scar tissue may have been caused by Anthony's elevated EBV and CMV levels.

Year Three

Infectious Disease Specialist:

At the end of our rope, we were referred to Dr. Bernstein. He listened as Anthony and I talked about the symptoms we noticed. He truly listened and then, told us that he felt it was probably Chronic Fatigue Syndrome. He wanted to run tests to rule out other illnesses. After the tests were run, he let us know that Anthony had elevated Ebstein-Barr Virus levels.

The doctor also gave us a definite diagnosis of CFS. After Anthony was diagnosed, he confessed, "I was starting to think I was going crazy." How horrible for a child to feel as if he has to carry the weight of the world on his shoulder.

The doctor didn't stop with that diagnosis. He continued to investigate and treat each symptom. What stands out the most about Dr. Bernstein is that he took the time to establish and cultivate a relationship with Anthony. He NEVER failed to make Anthony smile. No question Anthony ever asked him was beneath Dr. Bernstein to answer. He took the time to allow Anthony to process his thoughts so he could say what he really meant. It seemed their personalities were quite similar.

As time passed, Anthony even became playful with Dr. Bernstein. During one visit, Anthony decided to sit on the doctor's rolling stool. When Dr. Bernstein entered the examining room, Anthony stated, "Why don't you hop up on the table and let me see how you're doing." Dr. Bernstein looked shocked. He tried to proceed as if he hadn't heard, but a smile, and eventually a laugh, broke through.

I affectionately call Dr. Bernstein a "medical pit bull." He wouldn't let go. Whenever something didn't seem right, Dr. Bernstein dug deeper until he found an answer.

Dr. Bernstein was responsible for finding the Poland's Syndrome (a congenital disease) that Anthony has had since he was born. At times, when tests showed abnormalities, I could see how they troubled Dr. Bernstein. When tests and other specialists would confirm that symptoms were simply more "perks" from CFS, I could almost see the relief wash over him. Dr. Bernstein was the beginning of a turnaround for Anthony. He was the cornerstone in the medical maze.

The second time we were sent to the geneticist, it was to confirm that Anthony had Poland's Syndrome. This is a congenital disorder that wasn't detected until Anthony was already 14 years old. Poland's Syndrome is a disorder that can present abnormalities in the chest muscles (missing or underdeveloped) on one side of the body. On the same side of the body, a person may also experience webbed and fused fingers or hands/fingers that do not form completely.

Females have Poland's Syndrome more often than males. It usually affects the right side of the body. In Anthony's case, he's missing chest muscle and his chest cavity is smaller on the left side. The webbing between his fingers is barely noticeable unless someone is looking for it.

Hematologist:

Anthony was referred to a hematologist because a CAT scan revealed lymphadenopathy. He had too many lymph nodes and several were enlarged. The reason for that referral was to rule out cancer. Fortunately, no cancer was found.

This was probably the most brief doctor visit we endured. He told Anthony that he didn't need to be there, and that he regularly saw children in much worse shape than Anthony. We walked out of the examining room relieved at the doctor's lack of concern that it was some sort of cancer.

I still wondered why Anthony was experiencing the abnormality in his lymph nodes. After researching the term, I learned that the Epstein-Barr virus and the Cytomegalovirus can cause for lymphadenopathy. Anthony's blood work shows elevated titers for both of these viruses.

Physical Therapist Two:

It was again recommended that Anthony attempt physical therapy. We found a wonderful clinic and looked forward to making progress. During the phone interview, the receptionist exclaimed, "Oh, we have a wonderful program for Chronic Fatigue Syndrome!" After his initial evaluation, Anthony was given his own program. He lifted weights, stretched, rode the exercise bike, walked on the treadmill and used the hand bike. He completed his regimen. The unfortunate thing was that Anthony would fall asleep in the car on the way home and sleep the rest of the night. The next day, his pain levels would be unbearable.

He'd miss school for two days and then, it would be time for his next physical-therapy appointment. The cycle continued to repeat until I finally had to withdraw Anthony from physical therapy.

Physical Therapist Three:

I attended a CFIDS (Chronic Fatigue and Immune Dysfunction) conference, which was sponsored by the New Jersey CFIDS Association. I'll address the conferences later, but the most-important factor from the first conference is that I was blessed to have a moment to speak briefly with Dr. Peter Rowe after the conference.

I explained the vicious cycle of physical therapy, to crash back, to physical therapy. I told him that it couldn't possibly be therapeutic to continue in this cycle. He asked where I lived. Dr. Rowe happened to know of a physical therapist less than 30 minutes from me who had successfully treated some of his patients.

As soon as I arrived home, I called Aaron, the physical therapist. He spoke to me for approximately 30 minutes, answering all of my questions efficiently. He was patient with my concerns and fears. I was still apprehensive, but I made an appointment for Anthony for the following week.

I watched as Aaron evaluated Anthony. He tested each muscle group. He politely answered our questions and explained to Anthony everything he was doing.

Aaron's type of therapy begins as total manual therapy. Aaron's hands provided the resistance to Anthony's stretching. He stretched and rotated Anthony's joints and muscles. He spoke to Anthony about the pain posture of the body and how it could be counter-productive to the symptoms of Chronic Fatigue Syndrome. After the first real session, Anthony exclaimed, "Mom, I feel SO good!" I waited for a crash to follow. I'm still waiting for that crash, because it never came. Anthony actually got to a point of knowing when his body needed another session with Aaron. He looked forward to these appointments and ALWAYS left feeling better than when he went in. His pain levels decreased and he regained some of his strength and flexibility.

Aaron's gentle demeanor drew Anthony out. They joked and laughed. He'd finally met a man who could explain what was happening to his body and show him methods of relieving his symptoms.

Aaron's knowledge is endless. He worked with Anthony weekly and we gradually began to see a difference in Anthony's posture and pain levels. Improvement was all we were asking.

As Anthony's treatment progressed, Aaron formulated Anthony's home program. This program consisted of stretches that Anthony could perform in supine and prone (laying down) positions and/or sitting in a chair. Anthony was learning to manage his own body. He learned which stretches could help to alleviate which symptoms.

After speaking with Aaron about our dissatisfaction with Anthony's primary care physician, he offered to speak to some of his colleagues in reference to which doctors were knowledgeable about CFS and appropriate treatment. Aaron was responsible for giving us a ray of sunshine in a world that had become full of frustration and ridicule.

Pediatric Neurologist:

Dr. Myer evaluated Anthony to rule out any neurological disease. He stated that the evaluation was normal overall, but because of the cognitive deterioration of the past year; he suggested a neuropsychological evaluation "to ascertain Anthony's strengths and weaknesses in cognitive areas and to make sure he does not have a communication disorder of some sort." Once again, we were relieved to learn there was nothing out of order it this area.

Neuropsychologist:

Dr. C., the neuropsychologist tested Anthony to find out how Anthony was affected cognitively. I provided him with information about CFS before the testing. As with many of the children with CFS we've spoken to, Anthony's intellect was high, but he struggled in areas of short-term memory, attention, reading and writing. Dr. C. also felt that Anthony was preoccupied with his symptoms. Dr. C. also reported that the tests showed Anthony had difficulty with visual processing speed, verbal stimuli and possible dysgraphia. Dr. C. made some recommendations for Anthony's education. The results of these tests provided me with a concrete place to start in finding ways to help Anthony with his academics.

The difficult part about this testing is the length of time a child is required to perform. I made sure that Anthony got plenty of rest the day before so he would have the best chance of successfully completing it. It meant a lot to Anthony to do well on these tests. He wanted to get them completed before he "wiped out," so he refused to take the number of breaks he needed. He was exhausted and slept all of the way home.

Then, I helped him to his bed. When Anthony's teacher arrived, he was still exhausted and sleeping. He slept through the rest of that day and night. He also slept through the next day.

The hard part about testing these children is that the "tester" doesn't get to see the after effects of the testing. They note things like the child saying he's tired but not yawning. Since the child is fatigued all of the time, when would it be best for him to yawn? The last time I remember seeing Anthony yawn was before he got sick. It's something I hadn't even thought about until I saw the notes from the testing.

Internal Medicine Specialist:

Dr. Bowser is the doctor Aaron found for us. When I called to make the appointment, I was amazed at how much Karen, the office manager, was informed about CFS and FM (Fibromyalgia). She was supportive and encouraging. I was hopeful that this would be the doctor who could tie everything together. Anthony, at first, was reluctant to visit yet another doctor. He was tired and grumpy when we arrived for the appointment.

Dr. Bowser's new-patient-information form was the most precise and specific that we'd ever seen. It contained questions about every system in the body and its function. It contained a thorough family history. After completing the fourth page of the questionnaire, I realized we had answered questions we had never thought of.

Lawrence, the medical assistant, then led us, to the examining room. He went over the forms and asked us more detailed questions in relation to the answers we had given. There was no skepticism evident in the way he addressed us. He wanted to know more, and his demeanor encouraged us to let our guard down.

When Dr. Bowser entered the room, he asked even more questions as he examined Anthony. Within the first few minutes, Anthony was engaged in a playful banter with the doctor. Many questions flowed from Anthony, and many answers were given to Anthony in return.

Dr. Bowser provided comprehensive treatment (pharmaceutical medication and nutritional supplements combined). He boosted Anthony's immune system with nutritional supplements and treats the symptoms with prescription medications. Anthony's health began to change within the first month.

Dr. Bowser has helped us fight for Anthony's health and education. He is unstoppable. Whenever something troubles him, Dr. Bowser won't stop until he finds an answer. He accepts Anthony where he is physically and encourages him academically. He is an inspiration to Anthony because of the medical trials he faced in his own life. Dr. Bowser never gave up and he excelled. I think, through Dr. Bowser's example, Anthony realizes that he can also realize his own dreams.

Pediatrician:

I began calling doctors' offices with a list of questions. Does the doctor feel as if CFS is only of psychological origin? Is the doctor aware that children get CFS? Is the doctor aware that boys get CFS? Has he ever had any experience with CFS? I found a doctor who had the right answers to all of my questions. Dr. C. said he used to follow women's soccer. When an Olympic Women's Soccer Champion, Michelle Akers, was stricken with CFS, it piqued Dr. C's curiosity. He began researching the disease and also had another patient with CFS.

Dr. C. didn't try to blame the symptoms on Anthony or claim the symptoms were in Anthony's head. He accepted the diagnosis and was willing to consult with Dr. Bowser when necessary.

Since Dr. Bowser's office is an hour away, we needed a local doctor in case of an emergency. Once again, God provided for our needs.

Optometrist:

When Anthony began to experience an increase in his visual discomfort, I sought out an optometrist. I was familiar with Dr. D., because she treated me when the

Lupus affected my eyes. In the years I'd been diagnosed with lupus, nobody had ever addressed the visual component. I knew there was visual dysfunction in CFS; I needed to know what was specifically happening so I could help Anthony function.

Anthony had become resistant to reading even though he'd been reading since he was three years old. He said the words kept "jumping all over the page." He told me that he would get lost trying to follow from one line to the next. He told me that his eyes got blurry and hurt too much to read small print.

After a thorough screening, it was discovered that Anthony had an accommodative insufficiency. When trying to focus on a line of small print, Anthony's eyes would over focus. Then, his eyes overcompensate trying to adjust. This happens repeatedly when Anthony is reading, causing strain in his eyes, eye pain, headaches, etc. His eyes are also sensitive to light (especially fluorescent). I was told that Anthony had 20/20 vision. Before, I was told there was no problem because of Anthony's perfect vision.

There are other visual dysfunctions that are not found in a simple acuity test. It is important to follow this through when a child continues to complain of symptoms.

Treatments are available. It could be as simple as a special pair of glasses, or as much as vision therapy.

It's important to remember that the school eye exams are only checking for visual acuity (near-sightedness, far-sightedness, blindness, etc). They do not test for other types of visual dysfunction. If you feel your child is having visual problems, the child might need a specialist who is qualified to test for other types of visual dysfunctions.

Year Four

Neurologist #2

Anthony began experiencing moments of extreme disorientation. When Dr. Bowser heard this and noted unexplained bites on the inside of Anthony's cheeks, he hospitalized him to investigate the possibility of myoclonic seizures.

The attending pediatric neurologist was abrupt with Anthony and me. He demanded what method of diagnosis was used for Anthony's Carpal Tunnel. He spat, "Was his Poland's Syndrome diagnosed by a visual examination?" He cut me off after I told him it was found in an MRI and confirmed by a geneticist.

The doctor then asked what type of allergic reactions Anthony had with some medications. I barely finished answering the doctor when he told me which tests he was going to do on Anthony. The doctor abruptly turned his back on us and began walking out the door. As he was leaving, he looked over his shoulder and said, "It says here that your son has Chronic Fatigue Syndrome." I nodded. To this, he replied, "Do you REALLY believe he has this?" I said, yes I did and the doctor made a hasty retreat.

I went outside and called a friend for prayer. I knew the doctor didn't believe in CFS from the way he was acting. I also knew this from the way he saved mentioning CFS until last even though it was the first thing listed on the medical report. I told my friend that I didn't have the energy to fight. I only wanted to know for sure if Anthony was having seizures. I didn't want Anthony belittled because of someone else's ignorance! She prayed and when she was done, I went to my car and got a tape recorder in case the doctor wanted to become more belligerent. Still, I prayed that I didn't have to face that man while I felt so weak and vulnerable. We didn't see the doctor again that night.

One of the tests that was ordered was a sleep deprived EEG. BIG MISTAKE! In order for Anthony to stay awake, he was not allowed to take his medications (since they could make him sleepy). So, not only did Anthony have to stay awake all night, he stayed awake in pain! It was a miserable night. In fact, the only high point came when Anthony's friend Jamie surprised him and came to visit at the hospital.

When the test was completed, Anthony took his pain meds and immediately fell asleep. The doctor came in as Anthony slept and told me that the EEG did not pick up seizure activity. He thought it could have been some other things, but he wouldn't go into it with me. He insisted on only discussing it with Anthony's doctor.

The fall-out from that testing was that it severely disrupted Anthony's sleep pattern. It took several weeks to help his sleep pattern return to what was normal for Anthony.

Sleep Specialist

The neurologist recommended that Anthony be seen by a sleep specialist in order to have a sleep study performed. Anthony was not amused, and I was apprehensive.

Dr. P. was at first short with us. I tried to remain pleasant. Finally, I asked if Anthony was the youngest patient with CFS she had seen. She told me that Anthony was too young to have been diagnosed with CFS. I told her that that wasn't true as far as the CDC was concerned. She didn't argue with me. She just suggested a regimen to help Anthony get back on his regular sleep pattern again.

At the next visit, I brought literature about CFS in youth (including the CDC pamphlet). As we waited in the examining room, I noticed a copy of the CDC pamphlet on a shelf. This was encouraging. When Dr. P. entered the room, she was much more pleasant. She checked on Anthony's sleep pattern and scheduled Anthony's sleep study around Anthony's sleep cycle. When I asked if she was interested in some literature on pediatric CFS, she eagerly accepted it. She made a copy of the one handout I had no more of and kept the rest.

I think back on my initial internal response towards the doctor when she made her comment about Anthony being too young to be diagnosed with CFS. I truly wanted to lash out. I was frustrated by the fact that we had been in this battle for to long to still be facing the same misinformation. When I was tempted to react negatively, *"Be swift to hear, slow to speak and slow to anger; for the wrath of man does not produce the righteousness of God" ~James 1:19-20* floated around in my mind. I am grateful that the gentle admonition kept my tongue in line. Had I let my initial feelings of defensiveness and anger root, the opportunity would have been missed to raise awareness for another health-care professional.

Orthopedic Surgeon

Anthony has developed a Ganglion Cyst in his wrist. At this time, we are watching to see if the body will absorb it. Then, the doctor will decide what measures he may need to take in the future.

Occupational Therapist Evaluation

When the time came for Anthony to take the "behind-the-wheel" portion of his driver's education, the school occupational therapist and Anthony's case manager felt it was important for him to be evaluated by a specialist who focuses on the specific abilities and needs for a person with disabilities to drive.

The only appointment available, within our time constraints, was at 9 am. The rehabilitation center was 2 ½ hours away. We had to leave the house at 6 in the morning. As a back-up, my dear friend, Judy rode with us. It was very difficult getting Anthony up and moving this early in the morning. After I finally coaxed him into the car, he immediately fell back asleep for the duration of the trip.

He begrudgingly woke up and plopped into the wheelchair upon our arrival. We were processed in the intake office. We went over Anthony's patient information including medical history and medications. The case manager was kind enough to get water so Anthony could take something for pain. The concern on her face was genuine. She was sensitive enough not to draw too much attention to Anthony's pain. Instead, she gave us a general idea of what we would be doing as she led us to the office of the Driving Rehab Specialist.

As we waited for Anthony's specialist, another specialist (who also happens to utilize a wheelchair) drew Anthony into a light conversation. She expressed a desire to be the one who would work with Anthony if she didn't already have a client.

When Susan (Anthony's evaluator) arrived, she began taking general information from us about the disease and its symptoms. Anthony had his head in his lap as he listened to the questions. His head was still foggy from sleep. She was troubled by Anthony's seeming lack of alertness. She took a tough approach and tone with him that caused Judy to stiffen in her seat. I placed my hand on Judy's leg to reassure her that it was okay. Somehow, I calmly told the evaluator that Anthony was literally just waking up. She then asked me why I scheduled the appointment so early if I knew that Anthony didn't function as well in the morning. I explained how we had come to having an appointment so early.

Susan asked Anthony if he needed someone to read to him. He tried to explain his cognitive symptoms to her, but was not clear enough for her to understand. She then turned to me explaining that she needed to know how much Anthony's comprehension was affected. I explained to her that Anthony's comprehension was in fantastic shape. I backed that up with the fact that he had missed only one on the comprehension portion of the Virginia Standards of Learning test. In what seemed to be frustration and bewilderment, Susan moved Anthony to the first test.

The first evaluation was a test for divided attention. He completed the test without difficulty, and I could see that Anthony was waking up and the pain in his legs was subsiding.

The next group of tests evaluated Anthony's visual ability. He experienced some blurring, and I was able to explain that Anthony had an accommodative insuffiency that required him to wear glasses whenever he was reading for a sustained period. I restated that Anthony was literally just waking up when Susan first began to speak to him. I also reminded her that he had been in pain and was waiting for his medication to work. She then became concerned that Anthony's meds would have negative side effects. Anthony told her that it didn't cause drowsiness and she was satisfied.

Although Anthony forgot his glasses, his visual acuity tested at 20/15. Anthony's eyes were tested in range of motion, convergence, pursuits, near and far point fusion, depth and color perception and visual scanning. All tests results were scored within normal limits. As the tests progressed, it became a game to Anthony that he HAD to win. We laughed at his competitive nature. As Anthony's contrast sensitivity, visual perception and visual perceptual processing speed were tested, Anthony made it known to all that he was determined to get them all right! By the time these tests were completed, we all were laughing, and the cloud that had threatened to hang over the evaluation had dissipated.

When it was time for Anthony to take the driving test, we all went outside and saw the car he would be driving. Susan showed us some of the modifications that were available on the car, such as a left foot accelerator and a knob on the steering wheel. Judy and I stood on the sidewalk as we watched Anthony drive away. We were so obviously trying not to look obvious. It must have been comical to the casual observer.

When Anthony pulled back into the parking lot, he had an ear-to-ear smile on his face. As they got out of the car, he and Susan were clearly having a lively conversation. Anthony immediately shared the mistakes he'd made, but he also shared that he had been scared the CFS would prevent him from driving.

As we walked back into the building, Susan stated that she recommended that Anthony's only modification should be limits on the amount of time he spends driving (no more than one hour at a time). I reminded Susan that she didn't think Anthony could do it. We laughed as I told her how she looked at me like, "How could you be so cruel to do this to this poor child." She admitted that she was worried that he'd be too tired to test. I told her that I knew my son and wouldn't put him through any more than he could handle. We talked briefly about the disease and I asked her some questions about her facility. We then left for the long trip home.

At lunch, I expressed to Judy how thankful I was that I didn't jump when Susan was trying to get a response out of Anthony. Because of the cordial manner of communication, another professional ended up being made aware of CFS. To me, it's priceless.

Encouragement to physicians and other medical professionals:

We finally have peace with the treatment Anthony receives. We have confidence in the physicians. We have the "team" we could only have dreamed of a few years ago.

To physicians, I beseech you to make yourself aware of CFS and its symptoms. Please become informed about the various treatments. Please remain humble enough to acknowledge you cannot possibly know everything and then accept the fact that it's okay.

I accept the fact that anybody with a chronic illness may face times of depression. If you or your loved one is fighting depression, get him or her to someone who is qualified to diagnose and treat the depression. It is imperative that the counselor or psychologist is familiar with the difference in treating a major depressive disorder and treating someone who has secondary or situational depression. Anthony's depression was deep in the beginning stages of his illness.

His body had betrayed him. His cognitive skills had their own agenda, and the physician he turned to for guidance told him that he was only depressed and the rest was all in his head.

I am NOT advocating complete avoidance of possible psychological aspects. I am asking that those in the health profession do not forget the fact that there IS a physical aspect. I ask that all physicians, regardless of their knowledge of the CFS/FM, treat their clients with the same dignity they treat people with MS, cancer and other illnesses.

I remind everyone that until the 1950s, MS was considered to be a "hysterical disorder." There are specialists to evaluate and treat the physical symptoms. Mental-health professionals need to focus on treating the depression that might come as a result of the disease. I look forward to the day when a comprehensive CFS treatment center opens (providing physical therapy, occupational therapy, specialists, general practitioners, nutritionist, neuropsychologists, psychiatrists, psychologists). I can only imagine how great it will be when they all work together for total stabilization of body, mind and spirit.

We KNOW, at this point, there is no cure-all available. We are not looking to you to perform a miracle. We are looking to you to treat the symptoms, as best as you can, and be brave enough to walk with us through the storm.

You have the opportunity to truly make a difference in the lives of these children. The first step is only to truly listen.

Encouragement to Parents:

Don't be afraid to ensure that any physician or mental-health specialist acknowledges your child's diagnosis of a valid chronic illness before you take your child to his or her office for treatment. Find out if he or she is aware that children get CFS. Be sure that he or she is willing to learn about your child's disease. Inquire about their experience and knowledge of the difference in treating people with depression secondary to a chronic illness as opposed to people with major depressive disorders. If the answer to any of these is no or none, RUN, do not walk to the phone book and try again.

After one of Anthony's really bad days, one of my friends finally broke down crying. She told me that she felt like a hypocrite because she couldn't understand why Anthony had to be so ill. She felt like I was a "saint" for the way I was handling this. Let me confess to you all that I am in no way perfect. First of all, I have been in close battle for more than four years now. Still, I grieve because I didn't recognize the cognitive difficulties Anthony was having as his grades began to drop…even though I've worked with children with Learning Disabilities. There's no way I could have possibly known to look for them, but it doesn't stop the regretful feeling. I get sick of the battle and cry when I don't feel like fighting any more. I have cried because I don't have the answers to help my child. I cry when my child is in pain that ease. I cried when I had to carry

Anthony and banged his head on the dresser. I cried from the fear of fighting this battle without my husband. The ONLY saintly thing I've done is I have cried out to God. He has allowed my son to stay here on earth with me. He gives me peace that I don't understand. He gives me His strength in weakness. *God is my refuge and my strength, an ever-present help in times of trouble. ~ Psalms 46:1*

Chapter Six:
Medical Conferences

In the second year of Anthony's illness, I had the privilege of attending my first CFS conference in New Jersey. The New Jersey CFIDS Association sponsored this event. This conference was attended by people with CFIDS, physicians and parents of children with CFIDS. Some of the speakers were Dr. David S. Bell, Dr. Peter Rowe and Gloria Furst OTR/L, from the NIH.

Dr. Bell lectured about the effects of CFIDS on children. He shared with us the ratio of recovery he'd witnessed in his 15 years of research of this disease. He noted a list of symptoms. He allowed us to see an overview of the criteria for a diagnosis. We were informed of the other possible symptoms. For the first time, I realized that CFS has an impact on just about every system in a person's body. Dr. Bell's lecture was precise and left me with a better understanding of the battle my son was facing.

Gloria Furst spoke of the types of therapies used to attempt to rehabilitate the person with CFIDS. She showed us how to utilize Physical Therapy, Occupational Therapy, Speech Therapy, and Vocational Counseling in the treatment of CFS. Her lecture covered the recommended evaluation and therapies for the CFS patient. She also informed us about the process of graded therapy. This means a person with CFS is started out with a light load and gradually increases his therapy as his body can manage for a specific duration.

Dr. Peter Rowe spoke about Orthostatic Intolerance and CFIDS. He explained the relation of blood circulating volume to the increase of symptom severity when a patient is upright. I learned that increased activity is a risk factor. He also stated that improvement must precede reconditioning. He also recommended some methods of alleviating symptoms (changes in posture, increase of salt, increase of fluids). He then spoke of finding a 60 percent of patients who also had hyper mobility or Ehler's Danlos Syndrome. He named some medicines that raise the blood pressure such as Midodrine, Dexedrine (Zoloft, Wellbutrin) and Methylphenidate. Sodium, Fludrocortisone, Licorice Root, and Erythopoctin are used to increase blood volume.

One of the larger benefits I received from attending this conference was the occasion to actually see other people with CFIDS. I watched the young lady behind me wilt as the day progressed. She had to lie down on some chairs in order to attend even a portion of the conference. We lent her Anthony's manual wheelchair in order for her to make it to the restroom. Other people had to return to their rooms for the remainder of the conference.

We also met another child with CFIDS. We were actually in a place where EVERYBODY understood what Anthony was going through. I wanted to help everyone. My heart went out to the adults, because I knew, even though it's sad for children to have CFIDS, the children at least have their parents to care for and fight battles for them. I couldn't imagine what adults did to just function.

After the conference, I was blessed to have the opportunity to speak with Dr. Rowe for a few minutes. I explained to him how severely the physical therapy drained Anthony for days afterwards. I also told him that by the time Anthony's fatigue and pain levels returned to normal, it would be time for another physical therapy session. I told him that I couldn't understand how this could truly be "therapeutic."

From this brief conversation, our battle began to turn around. Again, thank you Dr. Rowe.

The next conference I attended was the Walk for Awareness in Washington, D.C. The threat of stormy weather changed the "Walk" into an indoor conference. It was informal and we had the opportunity to talk with several of the speakers. We spoke with Scott Davis Esq., Dr. Jacob Teitlebaum and Dr. Devin Starlanyl. We were allowed to ask them questions specific to our own situations.

From Dr. Teitlebaum, I learned about the use of comprehensive medicine (prescription and holistic) in treating CFIDS. Dr. Teitlebaum had CFIDS himself and managed to eventually recover. His books and treatments have helped some people recover to various degrees of function.

From Dr. Starlanyl, I learned about the symptoms of Fibromyalgia and Myofascial Pain. She was also kind enough to reach out to Anthony via email. She encouraged him to keep reaching for his dreams and offered ideas for ways he could do it. She stressed the importance of his education. She is a role model and an encouragement that these illnesses don't end our lives. She helped give him back the will and the drive to succeed.

From Scott Davis, I gained information about CFIDS/FM and social security. I have learned that sometimes people have to go on disability because of the debilitating effects of CFIDS and FM on their health and lives. I have been able to pass this information on to several adults I've met with CFIDS/FM.

Staci Stevens MA lectured about "Why Working Out Doesn't Always Work Out." Dr. Stevens is an exercise psysiologist (profession that looks at what the body does during exercise.) She emphasized that the focus should be on improving the quality of life and establishing a coping tool to help clients manage their illness. One statement she made has remained with me since I heard her speak. "If the patient doesn't recover, it's not a problem with the patient, it's a problem with the program." Finally! Eureka! Someone who doesn't blame the CFS patient for being sick! I couldn't wait to come home and share the quote.

This year, I went to another conference in New Jersey. Dr. Bell was again a featured speaker. He is now the chairman of the Chronic Fatigue Syndrome Advisory Committee. (the committee that makes recommendations to the U.S. Department of Health and Human Services) I was amazed at his intelligence and humility. This time, he focused on the autonomic nervous system and circulating blood volume. When I was speaking to Dr. Bell, he mentioned his desire to speak to school nurses. Since I was scheduled to hold a workshop in June, I invited him to come and speak. This change to the format of the workshop was quickly approved by the school system. I will be working with the teachers and their assistants on educational modifications and accommodations for specific symptoms of the illness. Dr. Bell will speak to the nurses, psychologist, counselors and special education designees.

I continue to go to every conference I possibly can. I encourage other parents, caretakers and children (as appropriate) to attempt to make it to at least one.

The feeling of swimming alone, against the current, will disappear. The number of other sufferers will awe you. The number of physicians who are truly trying to learn methods that will help you or your child will encourage you.

Chapter Seven:
Social Impact

Family:

I've learned from other mothers of children with CFS and women who suffer with this illness that men sometimes have a hard time dealing with seeing a person they love battle with CFS. This is, in no way, an attack on men.

Instinctively, we women seem to want to nurture when someone is ill. We, as mothers, are usually the ones who deal with the doctors and medical issues. To this day, when I don't feel well, laying my head on my mother's chest while she strokes my hair is blissful.

On the other hand, many men believe their job is to provide for their families and to protect all within their households. How perplexing it must be to have an enemy covertly come into your home and attack someone you love. On top of that, imagine an invisible enemy that comes in and attacks your wife or child that, at times, they sometimes find it impossible to function. You can't fight it. You can't fix it. You can't stop it. You can't save the one you love. All you can do is watch it happen.

We, as mothers, dive into researching and learning everything we can about the disease. We try to shield the children from the conflicts that arise with doctors, educators, insurance companies, etc. It's stressful to say the least. It's overwhelming if you have no support.

JJ, my husband had a double-whammy. He already had a wife with lupus. Now, his son has CFS. Doctors weren't helping. Schools weren't helping. He admitted he was terrified. I, at least, had much support from people all over the world via the Internet. I don't know, for certain, that my husband received support from anyone.

As this disease was beginning to disable Anthony, nobody, including Anthony, had a clue what was happening. He was slipping academically and his activity levels were severely decreasing. He tried valiantly to rise to the battle. As he started falling behind and failing to complete various assignments, chores and tasks, tension grew between him and my husband. JJ denied anything was wrong with Anthony because he "looked fine." Their close relationship hit rough waters for a while.

As the reality of Anthony's deteriorating health became increasingly evident, so did JJ's feelings of guilt. He didn't talk about it often. He just tried to make up for it.

The sad thing to realize is that, unfortunately, many marriages do not survive the onslaught of CFS… mine included.

Eventually, my husband left. He went to work one day and never came home again. I can't speak for him and won't even begin to try. We had other problems in our marriage. Finances were constantly being juggled. Honesty was lacking. All I am sure of is I don't have a moment to waste worrying about why someone else makes a decision he or she chooses to make. Whatever reason he chose to leave, it was not Anthony's fault for being ill. I'm not saying it didn't bother us. That would be a lie. The fact is we had no choice but to draw closer to God and each other. I allow Anthony to express his feelings. We pray together. We continue living. We still miss the other children from my husband's previous marriage. We allow ourselves to miss the family we had, but we don't allow it to consume us.

Maybe, because my husband left just a few months after September 11, it kept things in perspective. My husband didn't perish in a bombed building. He didn't go down fighting terrorists on a plane. He chose to leave. I had no control over his choice. My choice is how I decide to react to his choice.

This still left us to raise awareness about CFS to the rest of the family. My mother, at first, could not understand the decisions I was making for Anthony. She didn't understand how ill Anthony was. She didn't understand what was occurring cognitively with him and we ended up having a few heated discussions. This was especially painful for me because my mother is my best friend.

After Anthony was diagnosed, my mother read about the disease in order to inform herself. She asked questions when she didn't understand. She accompanied me to physicians' appointments. She joined me at the conferences. She is vigilant about Anthony's symptoms and health. She has become our shoulder to lean on and staunchest supporter, but she still has a tendency to "baby" Anthony…Then, again, that's what grandmothers do best.

My father had a hard time accepting the possibility that his only grandchild could be so terribly ill. He was scared and also resistant to learning about CFS. After Anthony and I moved back in with my parents, my father slowly began educating himself about the disease. He does a wonderful job of explaining to others what he knows about the effects of the illness. Over time, he has come to understand the coexisting symptoms like nausea and loss of appetite. The only problem is on the occasions of relapse; my father goes back into a bit of denial. I think it scares him to think Anthony could revert to the severity of when he first became ill. What I appreciate most is that I no longer have to argue to make a point about Anthony's health. It is no longer only solely on my shoulders to research CFS and inform the world. If something happened to me, I know my parents could quite capably carry the torch. I now feel that my mother and father are part of our team.

My brother knows very little about the disease. Sometimes, he innocently makes comments that hurt. He thinks Anthony is shy. If he only spent enough time around Anthony, he'd be surprised. I learned soon after Anthony became ill that I couldn't force anybody to learn about the disease. I love my brother regardless. He's the only brother

I have and the only uncle Anthony has.

Blessedly, our extended family has been remarkably accepting. They ask questions instead of forming opinions based upon assumptions. Neither phone call nor email is complete without inquiries about Anthony.

To those of you who are reading this for a loved one with CFS, I ask you to take the time to learn about this disease before you say something that may create a rift between you and someone you love that only God can heal. We need your love and support more than you could possibly imagine. We need your shoulder to lean and cry on. We need your hand to hold. We need your ears to listen. We need you to stand by our side (sometimes literally) when we walk into battles with schools, doctors, insurance companies, churches, etc. To those of you who are in the trenches with this personal battle, do not allow a seed to sprout a root of bitterness towards the ones whose ignorance prevent them from recognizing what your are dealing with. Focus your energy, instead, on those who will be supportive of your efforts and compassionate in relation to your weaknesses.

Friends:

Anthony, the once popular young man, became, within a matter of a few months, ALONE. I don't know if friends were afraid Anthony would die. I don't know if parents were afraid their children catching it. Were their lives so busy that they had no time for someone who could no longer keep up? I don't know. I do know that when school friends, friends from the neighborhood and church friends disappeared, Anthony was terribly hurt.

I don't know where we'd be if Anthony didn't have his incredible relationship with the Lord. He knew he was never truly alone. He clung to God and Jesus with everything he had.

I implored people to keep in contact with him. For two years, Anthony didn't see anyone besides doctors on a regular basis (at least once a month). People offered to take him on outings to the movies, but when he was too ill to go, they would go on without him. He was still left alone. We are so grateful for the times he was taken to the movies, but he so dearly craved one-on-one time with friends. From studying the history of the disability movement, I have come to understand how Anthony was so easily overlooked.

Our society, until very recently, was not conditioned to including people with disabilities in the community. When I was a young child, the children with limited abilities were kept separate from the general education students. We never had the chance to interact with them. I knew of the word retarded before I even knew what it meant. I only knew that it wasn't a nice thing to be called.

So, of course, we grew up not having a clue of the blessings these people can bring into our lives. Now, just when people think they have the politically correct labels and people sensitive language, here comes CFS, FM, NMH and many other invisible illnesses.

I won't waste a moment of my energy being bitter. Bitterness drives wedges instead of creating awareness. We HAVE to bridge that gap!

Religious Setting:

Anthony and I attended the same church for more than ten years. He was such an outgoing witness for Christ. He was humble trying always to give the glory to God. Anthony had been involved in almost every activity at the church and whenever the church doors were opened for an event, we were usually there.

One of his biggest hurts was the fact that once he became ill, in this setting also, he became entirely isolated. Because of his sleep pattern, he was unable to attend Sunday-morning services. When he became entirely bed bound, he was all but forgotten. He was reluctant to express the feelings he had because they went so deep. With gentle prodding, he released the hurt bit by bit.

As he released his hurt, I was forced to confront the bitterness that was threatening to overcome my innermost being. I prayed continually for God not to allow that seed to take root and wrap around my heart. My God, as always, was faithful and allowed me to look at the whole picture.

Our society (and most societies all over the world) has not been conditioned to expect people with limited abilities to be included as important and active members of our communities. In the past, people were encouraged to kill their "less than desirable" infants soon after birth. More recently, parents were encouraged to abort children that could possibly have defects. Parents were encouraged to put their children in institutions and get on with their lives.

These were all acceptable solutions. When I was a young girl in school, children with special needs were always kept in rooms down the hall away from the rest of the "normal" population. I can only remember real exposure to one girl with limited abilities from elementary through high school.

I don't remember ANY children with special needs in the churches when I was growing up. Now, just because the laws have changed, it doesn't mean people will miraculously know how to respond…even in the churches and temples.

I had to find a church that had evening services that Anthony could attend. I also wanted to find a ministry for children with disabilities. We found one seven minutes from my home. I was afraid for Anthony, but determined to try to find a church home for our family.

Anthony was welcomed at the new church. People seemed to accept him the way he was. Anthony kept his walls up for a while, but there were certain people who were persistent in their pursuit. The director of the accessibility ministry welcomed our family as a unit and went out of her way to help us feel secure in our surroundings.

Because Anthony was being spiritually fed and encouraged to serve, I was able focus on helping with the accessibility ministry. I attended the support group and helped when I was asked.

Anthony actually managed to help at Vacation Bible School this year! It was a physical sacrifice for him. We knew it would exact a payback. Anthony knew there was a little boy who needed him to be a buddy so he could go into the mainstream class. I weep when I look at the pictures.

Anthony would positively glow early on in the day. As the end of the day neared, he was obviously exhausted, but he pressed on.

Anthony became an immediate advocate for his buddy. He wasn't afraid to speak up and or come up with ideas to keep the child focused. He established his own reward/down-time system for the child. He was full of praise for the child. He still smiles when he speaks of the little boy.

Some people weren't sure how to adjust to a helper in a wheelchair. On the other hand, the people in charge of recreation figured out how to utilize Anthony's **abilities** when his group was outside. They looked past the wheelchair. They got to know him. They didn't assume that he was just shy. They pushed their way in and made him smile. The children, including Anthony's little buddy, made Anthony smile. His wheelchair was a source of fascination. They weren't scared of Anthony. They just talked to him…and talked…and talked. It was a learning experience for us all. I, now, more than ever, believe that God calls us to serve in whatever capacity we are able. We use whatever ability we have…even if all we can do is pray. God will bless us in the effort and bless others along the way.

When the church cancelled the evening services, once again, we were forced to find another church. I was shocked that after a year of Anthony attending, people in leadership would ask me why Anthony couldn't get up earlier or go to bed earlier so he could attend morning services. I was asked if I could still continue my ministry with the accessibility ministry in the days at this church while taking Anthony to another church in the evenings. It hurt, but I couldn't become bitter. I explained that if I was going to attend another church, I would have to be completely involved with that church. I couldn't sit on the fence.

After much prayer, I went to visit a small, older church in the community. It has been interesting to watch God draw the right people to Anthony. Nobody asks why Anthony keeps his head down. In fact, Ms. Carol has even given him his own pillow to get comfortable in church. God has given her the discernment to know when Anthony is having a rougher day than others. When she goes somewhere special, she doesn't fail to come back with something for Anthony. Ms. Carol calls Anthony a witness and inspiration for her. Anthony, on the other hand, asks me why she likes him so much. I know God had done this. God knew that if this love and commitment had come from someone who was a friend of mine, Anthony would have been guarded. So God sent a stranger to love Anthony so that Anthony could not doubt that God was watching over him and would send people to show His love in the human form.

The bitterness from before? Jesus has walked me through it. The bitterness has been replaced with a desire to help more churches reach out and include people with special needs. *That is why, for Christ's sake, I delight in weakness, in insults, in hardships, in persecutions, in difficulties. For when I am weak, then I am strong.* 2 Corinthians 12:10

We don't ask for the hardships, but we delight in the knowledge that our dear Father in Heaven will ever equip us to face the adversity asking us only to bear witness of his glory and faithfulness in all circumstances.

Co-workers

When Anthony first became ill, I had the support of my co-workers as I battled for his health and education. As time has passed, they became less tolerant of the many meetings and appointments that were necessary with Anthony's school, doctors and insurance company. Phone calls were not allowed. The final straw was when my supervisor actually hung up on my son's bus driver (calling to let me know she wouldn't be picking him up due to a surprise snow storm). This placed me in the position of choosing between my son and my job.

To me, it is amazing to see how people can be when they've never faced adversity. When a child is chronically ill, many things have to be balanced (insurance, doctor appointments, education, medications, therapies, etc). It is magnified when there is no spouse to help manage the care of the child. I pray that they are never in the position to have to juggle things so precariously.

I have truly become so weary of fighting. Yet, this became another area in which I was forced to fight. The environment became full of tension. Fortunately, I was able to transfer to another school, or I would have been forced quit my job.

Again, God has been gracious. I work for a woman who has illness in her family. I am overwhelmed by her compassion and understanding. She selflessly spurs me to fight when I need to, make calls when I need to and make appointments when I need to. Sometimes, she's more protective than I am! I have a haven in Peggy's presence.

I'm still not bitter. I pray for these people that they never reap what they've sown. More than anything, I wonder what other parents (more specifically single parents) do when trying to raise a child with a chronic illness and working at the same time. Do they quit their jobs? Do they take leave of absence (when the length of the illness in undetermined)? Do they hire a caretaker?

The books of Samuel in the Bible offered me great peace as I journeyed through this conflict. They give repeated examples of how someone, who is seen as lesser, is raised up and blessed by God for faithfulness.

Chapter Eight :
Where is the Silver Lining?

Before Anthony became ill, there was nothing he couldn't do. He could remember things from the age of three. He played any instrument that caught his interest and he played it well. His intellect was almost scary. He was a good athlete. He was outgoing and extremely talkative. He was popular. The girls were always looking at him, but he was too humble to notice. I was shocked when one young lady remarked after seeing him the first time, "Oooo, Ms. Shanon, you've gotta hook me up with THAT!" Anthony was thoroughly embarrassed. I was speechless.

Anthony seemed to be a magnet for children with attention-deficit disorders. My house was always full of his (very active) friends. His compassion and acceptance for and of others was remarkable. I can hardly imagine how Anthony must feel when he looks at the things he used to do with ease and then realizes that he has to struggle to even attempt them.

We wasted time. I wanted to help Anthony to return to the old Anthony. Anthony tried to return to the old Anthony. His body didn't cooperate and we both ended up feeling frustrated. When we came to the point of listening to his body, observing the signals it would give and modifying his day accordingly, he began to be able to do more. I guess we came to the point of acceptance.

We accept that this is who Anthony is right now. Once we learned to listen to Anthony's body and stopped fighting the symptoms, Anthony was able to do more as long as he paced himself. We accept the limitations of his body.

We focus on his abilities and allow them to take us in directions we never dreamed of. We accommodate for the limitations on his abilities. We understand that limitation does NOT mean halt. To us, it means finding other ways to accomplish a task. The blessing is the fact that we've become extremely creative. We live "outside of the box!"

Still, we prayed for a silver lining. We prayed for at least one friend for Anthony who would understand and accept the symptoms Anthony copes with. We prayed for this friend to like the same things that Anthony enjoyed. We prayed for a friend who wouldn't encourage Anthony to push past his limits. We asked God for a friend who would treat Anthony the same as he treats any other friend.

We had to trust. *Trust in the Lord with all of your heart and lean not on your own understanding. In all your ways, acknowledge Him and He shall direct your path. ~Proverbs 3:5*

Chapter Nine:
Safe Harbor in the Storm

After Anthony spent two years relatively alone and after much prayer, a boy who was in Anthony's kindergarten class renewed his friendship with Anthony. They got together one day in the late spring and have cultivated a unique friendship. Fortunately,

Jamie, the super friend lives caddy corner to our back yard. I marvel at how similar their personalities are. If I ask them a question, they will both respond with the same answer, same inflections and all.

I started by reminding Anthony to pace himself and limiting his time at Jamie's house. I then spoke to Jamie's mother explaining what had happened to Anthony's health. I also gave her the link to my web site in case she wanted to read more on her own.

Whatever concern I had at the beginning, was totally unnecessary. Jamie never encourages Anthony to push past his limits. On the other hand, Jamie doesn't pity Anthony either.

One of the funnier memories I have is when Jamie was digging a hole so we could plant my mother's new hibiscus plant. Anthony held the plant. I held the hose. We both watched Jamie dig the hole in no time flat. After we accomplished our task, we stood back marveling at our work.

They both started making wise cracks and I finally reminded them that I, the mighty mom, was the holder of the hose. They looked at me, stuck their chests out and said, in unison, "We are invincible to water." I turned the hose on them. Well, actually, Jamie hid behind Anthony while holding Anthony in place. Anthony got soaked! Later, that evening, we laughed at the obvious fact that Jamie would not show pity on Anthony. THIS was the kind of friend I'd been praying for.

As time has passed, the boys get together just about every day. On better days, Anthony climbs the fence and goes to Jamie's house. On not so good days, Anthony drags himself over the fence and "crashes" at Jamie's house. On bad days, Jamie will check on Anthony. If there is any virus going around Jamie's house, Jamie never fails to call and warn Anthony off a visit.

Jamie and Anthony have some mutual friends. They all get together at Jamie's house. He has also introduced Anthony to new friends. They have guy talk, listen to music, play games and just hang around. It's just what Anthony needed at the time he needed it most. They as close as any brothers I've ever known.

An added bonus is that Anthony has also formed a relationship with Jamie's parents, Heather and Donny. He calls them "Mom and Dad". He asked me if that offended me! I wanted to cry when I heard it because my child has NEVER felt close enough to other adults to even consider calling them "Mom" or "Dad".

The bottom line is, they just accept him. If he only feels well enough to come over, lie down and possibly fall asleep, they accept him. If he hurts too much to come to dinner, they bring dinner to him. If he's been too sick to come over, they lament about Anthony missing from the dinner table.

When my mother had a stroke, they willingly took care of Anthony so I could be at my mother's side. When I got sick with pneumonia, they were there as a haven for Anthony. When I have to go to the emergency room, they assure me that Anthony can stay as long as necessary.

I gave Anthony a surprise birthday party when he turned 16. Jamie was the first person who knew about it. He and his parents made plans to attend. I sent out the invitation to the people from the church he grew up in. The party was a week after Anthony's birthday, so he suspected nothing.

When we drove up to the "cookout", we were shocked to see about fifty people. Anthony didn't realize it was a party for him until people started singing. During the party, some people went swimming in the creek. Some were playing football. Some were playing other games. At all times, one or two people were with him. They learned not to crowd in on Anthony. They took turns spending time quietly with him. When Anthony realized Jamie and his family were there, he couldn't believe Jamie had managed to keep it a secret from him.

When Anthony got an award at school, Jamie managed to make it. Jamie's home is Anthony's sanctuary. He knows he's accepted no matter how he's feeling at that moment, what he's able or not able to do. These people ask for and expect nothing in return for their kindness. If there were an award for people who went above and beyond the call of friendship, they would be the winners.

Take note, people. Nothing is stopping you from being "super friends" except your willingness to step up. There IS a need for more people like Heather, Donny and Jamie. Who will rise to the challenge?

Chapter Ten:
The Impact of the "Waves" of CFS on Anthony's Education

The route to obtaining the right services, accommodations and modifications, was full of waves that threatened to sink us. The winds threatened to rip the sails off our vessel. Yet, we hunkered down and somehow, we've been able to weather the storm.

I include this segment because I want all to know that our children with CFS CAN be educated. They can experience success. They can also excel. All it truly takes is someone who is willing to learn about the disease, get to know the child and give help where help is needed.

I also include much detail so you can see the contrast of how ugly it can be when the committee doesn't know or refuses to really learn about the child's illness and how awesome it can be for the child when a team truly commits to working together for the benefit of the child.

Year One:

Anthony began his school year determined to make the honor roll. He planned ways he was going to be organized this year. He was also determined to get perfect attendance.

He had never done this because of injuries and illness. I don't know why he set this goal, but I supported him. He planned to continue to play in the band. He planned to run track in the spring. He had his whole year planned. Unfortunately, he had no idea of the storm that was going to rise up in his life.

By the late fall, the problems with his digestive system had begun. He did his best to hide it, but began missing days of school. He forgot to turn in papers from homework. He forgot to turn in class work. He forgot to do homework. After he was hospitalized, we knew that he didn't have the strength to return to school. He was wiped out. His legs

were weak. His digestive system was unpredictable. He had numerous appointments with various doctors.

He was placed on homebound schooling for the remainder of the school year. Enid, a friend and teacher with whom I worked, offered to come to the house and teach Anthony for homebound. She had previously been Anthony's fifth-grade teacher. It must have torn her up to see him so ill, but she worked out a way to teach him at his best time, and Anthony was able to progress to the eighth grade.

There were problems with the school getting assignments to her, but she stuck it out fighting the battle and shielding me from the mayhem. Anthony longed for his friends from school and the neighborhood, but he couldn't keep up with them. With physical therapy and a treatment plan from the gastroenterologist, we naively felt we would soon be out of the woods.

Year Two:

Anthony began the new school year with the intentions of returning to normal life. He was an office assistant instead of taking P.E. I spoke with his new team of teachers, explaining Anthony's history of health issues. I asked them to let me know if they saw anything that raised flags.

He was doing well in art. He was surprised at the amount of Spanish he remembered from his younger years. He tried to keep up with schoolwork. He was so excited about the new school year. I, on the other hand, was apprehensive. He still didn't seem "well" to me. He tried so hard to be normal.

Again, he started missing school. I spoke to his guidance counselor about the possibility of placing him on homebound again, but Anthony insisted on trying to attend school. As his health began deteriorating, I was able to persuade him to attend school only half days. I began getting calls at work from the guidance counselor. The teachers were coming to her with concerns about Anthony's health. He arrived for one class, went to lunch and then would "crash." We were in the middle of the hunt for a diagnosis. He was frequently taken to the doctor (sometimes at the school nurse's urging) with swollen lymph nodes, pain, and weakness and extreme fatigue.

I later learned that some others at the school were trying to carry out a chintz (truancy) petition against me. We had no diagnosis. At one point, depression was the only thing the doctor would use to support Anthony's homebound status.

That diagnosis (though we didn't like it) was enough to buy us time until we could find a diagnosis. Once we received the diagnosis, I asked for a child-study meeting to determine which services would best fit Anthony's academic needs.

Child Study:

At the initial meeting, I explained the disease and symptoms to the committee. I thought, with my experience in working in special education, with the training I was required to take, with what I knew about the IDEA, that it would be a smooth transition. I submitted some recommended modifications. Even with the doctor's diagnosis and recommendations, I was still greeted with skepticism. I was told that my son would "never" get some of the suggested modifications because of high testing scores from the years before he became ill.

I asked that Anthony be evaluated to find out if he qualified for special education services. Instead, I was encouraged to get services from Section 504. They even had the form ready to sign for 504. *Personally, I feel that Section 504 meets the needs of people in short-term limited ability. I do believe Section 504 can work for children with CFS who are in remission or have at least made a substantial improvement.* I told the committee that I would not sign a 504 until Anthony was tested to see if he qualified for Special Education Services under the IDEA. The climate in the room changed to antagonistic and cold. I was asked by the school psychologist "Why do you WANT your son to be labeled Special Education?" I told that no parents WANT that for their children, but if it takes a label to get him the services he needs, label him. My joke is: I don't like labels. In my lifetime, I've been called colored, Negro, black and African-American and I've never been to Africa in my life…and nobody has ever taken my vote! Finally, the committee relented and someone left the room to get consent forms for the evaluation process to begin. I was asked to get copies of the doctor's notes and submit them to the committee. Once the form was signed, I stood to leave and thanked the committee. The psychologist sneered, "We need to rule out the possibility that this isn't just a psychological issue, first!" I was shocked, overwhelmed, and bewildered. I was only in the eye of the storm. The worst was yet to come.

My new friend, Mary Robinson recommended I buy a copy of the book, <u>A Parent's Guide to CFIDS: How to be an Advocate for Your Child.</u> (written by Dr. David Bell and Mary Robinson). I downloaded the IDEA on my computer. I contacted an advocacy center. I began keeping a journal of **all** contact between the school and myself. Mary and Michelle, with their professional experiences with Special Education and CFS, came along beside me and talked me through each step of the battle that I had no idea was approaching.

Evaluation Process:

It seemed that every time the committee school psychiatrist and I spoke, we'd end up in an argument. The most insane argument was over how much time she needed me to allot for Anthony's testing. She explained the importance of this "I.Q." testing. I tried to explain the importance of planning and pacing in order to prevent Anthony from crashing. She wouldn't tell me how much time it would probably take.

Somehow, this turned into a 10-minute argument! I told her that I needed to know in order to adjust Anthony's schedule of doctor appointments, rest, counseling and testing. She wanted Anthony rested so he could do well on the test. I told her even if he was rested before the testing, she might not get an accurate score because of the fluctuations in his symptoms.

At this point, she asked me if I was saying I didn't want Anthony to do well on the test?! I realized we were getting nowhere, and I asked her why we ware arguing when we were supposed to be working together to help the same child! I finished off the conversation telling her that she was unbelievably and unprofessionally rude. I explained that no matter what professional certificates she had, I expect her to speak to me with the respect of one adult speaking to another. She said nothing. I said goodbye and hung up. A co-worker, who was in the room during the conversation, encouraged me to document everything that had just happened in the conversation. From that moment on, I stopped speaking to the school psychiatrist without another person present. Instead, I began writing all of my communications to the committee.

Anthony's psychological testing ended up being broken into two days (two hours each day). Before the second test date, Anthony developed a sinus infection and had to be placed on antibiotics. We informed the school psychiatrist that he was fighting the infections and on antibiotics when she took him to be tested.

103

On several occasions, I asked the committee to test Anthony for specific cognitive difficulties. They never did. His psychological report consisted of self-report depression tests. After all of the arguing, my son's I.Q. was never tested.

The teacher who administered the educational testing was pleasant, but it was obvious that she too disbelieved that CFS was a true medical disorder. She planned to break Anthony's testing into two days. On the second day the testing was scheduled, we showed up with Anthony, and she wasn't in school that day. She had forgotten about

Anthony's appointment and taken the day off. Nobody called to cancel our appointment. No apology was ever given.

Both the psychological and educational evaluators kept Anthony longer than agreed, despite being informed about the fatigue factor and pay back.

The social worker took information about Anthony's social history. Out of everyone on the team, she was the only one who treated us kindly. I couldn't tell if she was or wasn't a skeptic from the way she treated us. There was just something different about her from the others.

I asked to receive copies of the reports 48 hours prior to the meeting (as provided in the IDEA). I didn't receive the reports within the required time frame. When we read over the reports, it was obvious that our instincts were right.

Neither the psychological, nor the educational reports mentioned that Anthony was diagnosed with anything. It was known at that time that Anthony was diagnosed with CFS, Asthma and Poland's Syndrome. When Anthony performed well on a test, the evaluators attributed it to Anthony's intellect. When he performed less well because he was feeling poorly, the evaluators claimed it was because "Anthony put forth little effort" or "had less interest in it."

The psychiatrist had spent some of her time calculating the number of days Anthony missed from school between the first and eighth grades. He had missed 157 days (not including homebound services.) She didn't mention the fact that these absences were excused and most of them for medical reasons. She claimed Anthony's grades from the past weren't up to his potential due to his lack of effort. I'm not sure how she came to this conclusion because she'd never spoken to his former teachers.

She included statements attributed to Anthony that Anthony told me weren't true. After reviewing the reports, Anthony proclaimed that he was going to the meeting to speak for himself. Otherwise, he felt, they would say I was making things up. At this stage of the illness, Anthony was up one to two hours a day. He felt this meeting was important enough to expend all of his energy. It took a lot of extra willpower for him to make it to the meeting. Somehow, he valiantly rose to the challenge.

Eligibility Meeting:

When some of the committee members realized Anthony had accompanied me to the meeting, they sent someone to ask if I wanted to leave Anthony in the waiting room for the beginning of the meeting and then bring him in later. I firmly responded that it was Anthony's meeting and he had the right to be there.

Anthony slumped with his head in his lap, exhausted, while the reports were read to the committee. He poked me in the leg each time something was read with which he disagreed. I wrote them down to help him recall the topics he wanted to address.

When the committee chairwoman, Mrs. P., asked Anthony for his comments, he sat up and addressed each point on the list. He was assertive and respectful. I was proud of him. He, for the first time, spoke out as his own advocate.

The psychiatrist also stated that Anthony told her that he "works some afternoons at the Animal Rescue League." Anthony told her that he's never worked at a job in his life. He explained to the committee that he sometimes went to my friend's house who did animal rescue and played with the animals (pet therapy recommended by counselor). She sheepishly said she "must have misunderstood." I explained to the rest of the committee that Anthony was battling a sinus infection and headache the last portion of the testing and even though I had informed those who administered the test, they made no mention of that fact in their reports.

Instead, one made a comment in her report that, "he alluded to pain." Anthony made it clear to the panel that when he says he's hurting, he's really hurting. In their reports, they tried to deny that Anthony's hands hurt because he rolled a pencil on the table and manipulated a stapler and paperclip.

Anthony explained to the panel how it required different muscles and hand positioning required for writing as opposed to rolling a pencil back and forth on a table. Anthony exclaimed, "How many more do we have?" "I'm about to blow out." The psychiatrist stated the response came because the tasks "appeared to be less intriguing to him." In reality, what Anthony was telling her was that he'd done just about all he could.

What upset me most about the reports was the fact that they were supposed to be impartial and thorough evaluations. I believe when an examiner is biased, he or she should remove herself from the position of evaluator.

In these reports, Anthony clearly complains about his eyes, hands and head aching. He clearly mentions cognitive problems, but those comments were attributed to him not trying or wanting to try. His listening comprehension scores were on a fourth-grade level and the comment was made, "He said he was having difficulty remembering information from even the simplest passages. Due to his headache and what appeared to be lack of effort on this subtest, results are not a valid reflection of Anthony's listening comprehension." I don't know what these assumptions were based on. To me, these were indicators that something was wrong. To the evaluators, it was all Anthony's fault and in Anthony's control.

Had these people not had previously determined biases; we could have really made some strides in aiding Anthony in the educational process.

The homebound teachers, Dr. Gates and Mrs. Maddox stuck with us throughout the school year. They truly took the time to observe Anthony regularly and reported to me any concerns they had. They learned that reading (or trying to read) caused Anthony's frustration levels to elevate. We had to establish a method for Anthony to communicate his frustration, pain and fatigue levels. For instance, at the start of each session, Anthony was asked, "On a scale of 1-10, where are your fatigue levels, pain levels, cognitive fogginess." If they noticed Anthony going downhill, he could be asked these questions at any time during his instruction. If he, at any time, reached above a seven, stopping the instruction or changing the modality of instruction was considered. If his levels were eight or above; instruction was stopped.

The homebound teachers read about the disease. We swapped ideas for techniques that could possibly be helpful and we devised new ways to help Anthony learn. They shared what they observed in the months of teaching Anthony with the committee. I was impressed by how much they had learned over such a few short months.

Boldly, they stood up for Anthony's needs, even though what they were saying seemed to be contrary to what the committee wanted to hear.

When the committee was deciding what services Anthony was or was not authorized to receive, again, the psychiatrist balked. I finally asked her what her aversion was to CFS.

Her response was that "CFS is an elusive diagnosis." I retorted that it was an exclusionary diagnosis. I explained that many doctors are seen and many medical tests are performed before a diagnosis is given. It is not an easily given, throwaway diagnosis.

She told Mrs. P. that she had sent me a letter asking for authorization to speak to Anthony's doctor and I had never responded. She also complained that when she called the office that morning that she was informed that I said I "would not authorize" her to speak with the doctor. I explained to the committee that three days before she even wrote that letter to me, Anthony had an appointment with the doctor. I was then informed that she had already called his office and tried to speak to him without my authorization.

She tried to excuse her actions by claiming she was, "only looking for general information." I reminded her that she could have called any other doctor in the town to obtain "general" information. Then, she claimed she only wanted to know if EBV had been isolated in Anthony. I informed the committee that Anthony had elevated levels of

EBV and I would have the doctor fax copies of that report to the school. I also told them that I had no problem with someone else on the committee speaking with the doctor (I even offered the cell phone) but I would NEVER authorize the school psychiatrist to speak with my son's doctor.

I asked her why she was so focused on the EBV. Somewhere, she got the idea that the EBV was imperative for a CFS diagnosis. I informed her that not all people with CFS have elevated EBV levels.

She wanted to delay the decision until after Anthony's appointment with the hematologist (due to lymphadenopathy). Fortunately, the Mrs. P. took up that argument and I was able to relax. She had truly listened to all Anthony and I had to say. She had looked at the documentation I had provided. Obviously, she stood up for the child.

After a lengthy and heated meeting, Anthony was finally approved for special education services under the OHI (Other Health Impaired) classification criteria.

IEP Meeting:

We attended a meeting to construct Anthony's IEP. We met with the Assistant Principal from the high school Anthony would attend. She immediately began reading the information I provided about the disease. She spoke to Anthony without skepticism. When unsure, she asked questions instead of making assumptions. This was truly a meeting focused on Anthony's needs. Several suggestions were made. The educational evaluator seemed to change her attitude.

Unfortunately, no matter how cheerful and supportive she appeared to be at this meeting, we were still leery of her. I don't think I would or could ever trust her with issues concerning my son's welfare again. We made plans for his ninth-grade year. We prayed that this would be a better year for him.

I have mixed emotions about the interactions we had with this committee. I am so proud of Anthony for speaking up. On the other hand, it makes me sad that he even had to. How does it make a child feel to have the people in authority form a bias against something that is hurting and impeding the child physically, emotionally, socially and academically? Do these people realize they lose the respect of these children? How can a child be expected to respect someone who puts things in an official document that are untrue? If Anthony ever sees any of these women again, he has no choice but to be respectful in his actions. Their images and characters, in his eyes, are terribly tarnished.

2001-2002 School Year

Anthony started this school year full of hope. He started out going to school for one class a day. He developed friendships. Leah, his teacher was attentive to his needs. Soon after the school year began, the bus didn't pick him up. By the time the error was realized, Anthony was so ill that he couldn't remember his address or how to get to the house. He missed a week of school. Then, his body was not able to recover.

On paper, his IEP looked wonderful. We had to have several meetings in order to help the teachers understand how to make the modifications and exactly what his needs were. Although he started school, his homebound services were not established. I called two weeks prior to school starting to inquire about the process and was told I wouldn't hear anything until after the first week of school. By the time a teacher was finally hired, we were into the seventh week of the school year. Apparently, the previous school hadn't passed the information on to homebound services after the IEP was established. I finally had a parent advocate sit with me in the meetings. I needed someone I could bounce ideas off. I needed someone to tell me if my desires were unreasonable. It had become such a stressful situation.

Martha, the advocate, was a source of moral support. I wish I had known that parent advocates were in existence when I fought with the middle school. Martha was instrumental because of her history of working in special education. She was also up-to-date on what services were available and what my son's rights were.

The school year did not progress as smoothly as we had hoped. Three of the teachers jumped on the bandwagon. Other teachers refused (literally) to make some of the accommodations and modifications for Anthony listed in his IEP. The bad part was these teachers taught Anthony's worst subject. One told me, "None of my students get study guides!" Even after me drawing her attention to Anthony's

IEP, she still never sent them. They worked against the case manager instead of with her.

Anthony's homebound teachers, Elaine and Linda, were determined to help him catch up. They also listened to him and allowed him to tell them when he had done all he could. They recognized that he was not a quitter or malingerer. They acknowledged that when Anthony said he couldn't, he truly couldn't. They also learned how to get him to express where his pain, fatigue and cognitive levels were at any given moment. They walked by my side and never gave up. I'm grateful. What they have done for my child can't be taught in books. No college course prepared them for this. It's just who and what they are.

Anthony's Algebra teacher, Linda, decided to come over and catch him up with the class. She played a big part in getting him to really trust an adult from the school again. He laughed. He smiled. He enjoyed learning again. I ended up sitting up at night making study guides, reading to him, helping him with his homework typing for him. I would do research on the disease when Anthony was done with his lessons. Then, I'd sleep for a few hours and get up to go to work helping other children. I was exhausted and it was taking a toll on my Lupus. One of the final straws came when the Standards of Learning tests were to be taken. Anthony's homebound teacher was informed on a Friday that the tests would begin the following Monday. She and Anthony crammed all weekend (on her own time). Since homebound services had begun seven weeks late, they had to review everything he had learned and touch on everything he should have learned up to that point.

Anthony was exhausted but wanted to do well on the tests. He pushed himself past pain and fatigue until the testing was done. He never made it back to school.

Conflicts and omissions continued throughout the school year. By May, I contacted the Department of Education (DOE). They asked if I had spoken to everyone on the chain of command. They asked if I had documentation. Along with my letter of complaint, I sent a copy of Anthony's Educational Journal, message notes, emails, written correspondence, and tape recordings of meetings. Anthony managed to catch up in all of his subjects except for the class in which the teachers refused to make the accommodations. He had to take the class over the summer and he obviously resented it. He didn't go to summer school because he did anything wrong; he had to go because of wrong choices someone else made.

The DOE contacted the school system about my complaint. They drew attention to specific state and federal violations. To elaborate, they directed the school system's attention to my notes. The school system was given a specific amount of time to respond to my accusations. After the DOE contacted the school system, I was contacted and asked to come in to see if we could work out the differences. Wisely, Mrs. P. was selected to deal with me. I trusted her and knew we could try to work things out. I knew she would do all in her power to insure that this agreement was followed through.

2002-2003 School Year

This year was the best since Anthony became ill. As agreed with Mrs. P., we met with all of the subject teachers about Anthony, his illness and academic needs. The new case manager took the time to make herself aware about CFS and then got to know Anthony. She has done everything in her power to get Anthony whatever he needed.

The first grading period, he was allowed to attend school for one class a day in his wheelchair. Since mathematics is his best subject, it was decided he would attend the

geometry class at the school while taking the rest of his classes (keyboarding, English, and biology) in a homebound setting. Anthony excelled and his health didn't suffer dramatically. The Geometry teachers applied some of Anthony's accommodations and modifications to the rest of the class, such as using different colored chalk and paper.

They were excited about finding new ways to help Anthony learn. They were aware of his intellect and delighted when they found ways to help him demonstrate his knowledge.

We decided to add another class to his school attendance.

He attended Geometry and had lunch in a quiet place. Then, he went to Driver's Education. Again, there were no real problems with the accommodations and modifications.

When Driver's Education ended, we substituted English as his second subject. His English teacher was made aware of Anthony's needs and she worked to help Anthony successfully complete the course requirements. I worked with Anthony to keep him caught up. I, then, got a bad case of pneumonia. His English teacher, on her own time and asking for nothing in return, came over to the house to help Anthony stay caught up in English. Her true concern over Anthony's welfare brought me to tears. I had finally arrived at a point that no longer had to worry about Anthony while I was at work and he was at school.

Anthony was assigned a paraprofessional to help him with Driver's Education and English. Whenever he talks about her, he smiles. She makes him laugh. Evidently, she's just the right amount of joyful and silly that she can make him respond. The only negative thing that happened was one day; Anthony didn't make it to the bus. Anthony was more worried about me being mad at her than missing the bus. He said she was crying and kept apologizing. He was concerned. I wrote a letter to her letting her know that I wasn't angry with her. I told her it meant more to me that she could always make Anthony smile. It meant more to me that she never left Anthony's side until he was picked up. She didn't abandon him out of avoidance of my reaction. That was priceless.

Anthony began having severe pain with attempting to type. We figured this was a progression of the symptoms. We dropped keyboarding class. Anthony decided to take Art classes. Of course, people were shocked at the idea of homebound art because it had never been done.

Surprisingly, his new homebound teacher majored in Art in college and was willing to teach Anthony Art at home. He had to complete his art and driver's education classes over the summer.

I wanted to provide Anthony with enlarged font textbooks since it was in his IEP. The committee brought in the vision specialist. I also wanted Anthony to be allowed to use voice recognition software, so the assistive technologist was also added to the team.

The Vision Specialist wanted proof from a doctor that Anthony had a visual dysfunction since the school nurse testing said he had 20/20 vision. The AT jumped in telling the team that her daughter was a "case study for the NIH" and they don't give her enlarged font books. She talked about the specific testing and guidelines that have to be followed before a Visual Disability is even considered. I then had to ask three times (amid interruptions and debate) before I was given a copy of the criteria. I got a copy of the AT report at the meeting, so I was already on guard. The report on the 45-50 minute observation consisted of reporting on Anthony using scissors, using a pencil/pen to take notes, and a comment Anthony's classmate made when he offered to help Anthony to his wheelchair. The classmate said, "Anthony, you've got to get out of your black mood." She also felt it was okay for Anthony to be dependent on a scribe instead of utilizing software that would allow for future independence with the writing process. She made comment that she is concerned about Anthony's "mood swings" and wants the team to stay

117

aware of the "lows and highs." She talked about Anthony wearing black when he was feeling "low."

By this time, my frustration level was high. My son wears black when he's naked! I agreed we'd meet again after I got Anthony to doctors who could give yet, more documentation on Anthony's limited abilities. It was frustrating to come into a meeting with people who truly have no clue what's transpired in the two years since we spoke and have them make psychological assumptions about my son that the teachers who see him daily are NOT in agreement with. More than that, it is highly insulting for someone to tell a black person that the color black has to represent something negative all the time. It is definitely not politically correct. Actually it borders on the archaic. The meeting ended with the team agreeing to a complete evaluation series on him and I was to make appointments with physicians.

The teachers were shocked when they read the report. This time, it's the teachers who are willing to work as a team and the related services staff who are not. We met again after the evaluations. They figured out the areas that are cognitively difficult for Anthony at the moment. I provided the physician's diagnosis of Carpal Tunnel and Raynaud's Syndrome. I provided the optometrist's diagnosis of accommodative insufficiency.

Neither were enough to receive services. The AT mentioned that she had spoken to the person in charge of vision at the DOE and "she said she would NEVER recommend enlarged font books for a child with CFS." If this person said this, I hope they realize that they cannot group all children with CFS and deny visual services just because the child she came in contact with previously didn't need it. Again, the AT started talking about her daughter and I finally blew. The bottom line was, "This meeting is not about your daughter. It's about Anthony." She got frustrated and left the meeting.

I asked for prior written notice and finally got it. They thought it would be enough to tell me. I can never relax that much. I managed to get information about a program from a man at Voice Solutions in California. I then managed to get the program at a special rate.

My next step was to apply to one of the foundations for Anthony's dream of a laptop. I purchased the program and waited for the laptop. The Sunshine Foundation approved Anthony's laptop request. Gateway computers provided the laptop to Anthony's specifications. All they asked in return was for a picture of Anthony with the laptop. Over the years, that laptop has seen much use. When Anthony is stuck in the bed, the laptop is his best friend. I've learned that God will make a way for anything He has for you. He will always give you what you need, but sometimes, you also end up with the desires of your heart.

I dropped the battle with the Vision and AT specialists, free to return to it if necessary. I focused on Anthony's education and health. We devised other ways around those specific needs. If they become more of a problem to Anthony, I will take up the banner again.

At the end of this school year, Anthony received an award for a 3.5 or above GPA. He also received the award for the highest GPA out of 5 geometry classes in the school. He didn't inherit it from me. It was all of his hard work that got him that Geometry grade. It was also the blessing of the entire team working together. Even though some of his classes were homebound, the school-based teachers knew who he was and had a relationship with him. They knew what his needs were and were dedicated to seeing that they were met. They did this, not because they were worried about my response, but because they were dedicated to their student. I must tell you that I did write a letter of apology to the AT. It dawned on me that I had been so offended by the "wearing black must mean you're depressed" line of thinking that I shut her out. All I can do is hope she had no knowledge of how offensive what she had said truly was. I took responsibility for my anger. We have not been in contact over my son again, nor do I think we ever will, because she's not a person he's comfortable with anymore.

Regardless, that was one grudge I had to let go. This year was, overall, an outstanding year. There are awards (with a parent's nomination) the special education committee offers to people who go out of their way to help children with special needs. I nominated three of Anthony's teachers and his paraprofessional. I also nominated his case manager. They were surprised with their well-deserved awards. That was the best I could give after all that they've done. These will be the teachers that Anthony will, in the future, come back to in order to thank for helping to turn his life around. I believe in advocating for your child when something is going wrong. I also believe in acknowledging the hard work of others when things are going right. The hardest skill to learn is to not hold what one team has done wrong against the next team to come along. It's hard to trust when you feel your child has been wronged. Hopefully, you will be able to work through the differences and have the whole team work together, evening out the glitches amongst the whole group.

2003-2004 School Year

Anthony began the school year taking algebra and chemistry at school. He took English, history and art as homebound services. We met with all of the teachers (except English) at the beginning of the school year. They were able to ask questions and join the web site I set up for communication between Anthony, the school and me. It is a private site where the teachers can learn about the symptoms specific to Anthony. All of the teachers joined.

The school provided a mask for Anthony to wear during the use of chemicals in chemistry classes. Anthony adored his algebra and chemistry teachers. He came home daily with new and interesting things he'd learned.

The unfortunate occurrences of Anthony having health new health issues and the flu appearing in almost epidemic proportions required the removal of Anthony from school because of his compromised immune system. Anthony missed his teachers, but continued to receive his homebound services.

Again, we were having problems getting his modifications met in his English class. I couldn't make the teachers understand that the modifications and accommodations were imperative for Anthony to have success in English. Once again, we had to have frequent meetings to address how Anthony's needs were not being met. We couldn't have made it without his homebound teacher who was willing to advocate for Anthony. She took up the fight and if she found a problem with the work she was given, she faced the teachers to straighten it out.

2004-2005 School Year

I can't believe my son is finally a Senior! I prayed that this year would be the perfect year for Anthony. It was decided that Anthony would attend all mainstream classes (not collaborative/inclusive classes). His one-on-one paraprofessional would attend his classes with him to act as a scribe and reader as Anthony needed.

On orientation day, I took Anthony to the school to meet all of his teachers. The case manager gave each of the teachers' folders containing information about children with Chronic Fatigue Syndrome. I look forward to this being a smooth and memorable year for my son.

Well, the school year is ½ over and it has not been a smooth year. Again, we face educators who know nothing about the illness and are not making an effort to learn about it. At meetings, one teacher made a comment about trying to "push" Anthony. Another made a statement about "like normal kids."

I am frustrated because I don't want to fight this battle once again, but as you read this book, forward I am going.

Educators, you must recognize that sometimes (if not most times), the parent knows their child best. You must acknowledge that when a new illness is found, the parents usually *know* the difficulties the child is facing, and they look to you for guidance in how to best serve their children's academic needs. You, as educators, will need to make yourself aware of the symptoms of new illnesses if you are going to fulfill a child's academic needs. As more children are diagnosed with invisible disabilities, more accommodations, strategies and modifications will have to be learned. It becomes easier to do when you think about how you'd feel and what you would want if you woke up tomorrow morning not being able to do what you used to. How would you cope? Would you be angry? Would you be frustrated? Would you want someone to tell you, "It's only depression?" Would you want to be isolated? Would you want people to act as if you were just lazy? Would you want to be left alone to try to figure out how to make your brain and body function right again?

I believe the answer to all these questions is, "No!" These children need educators to listen to what they have to say. They need educators to communicate with them about their symptoms. They want educators to help them figure out ways to realize their dreams despite the illness. They don't want pity. They want to be treated with dignity. They want people to take the time to understand their illness.

Chapter Eleven:
The Life Preserver

Before Anthony became ill, I was the perfect Internet illiterate. As time has passed, I have become the Internet Queen!

Initially, I threw myself into researching on various search engines. I consumed every piece of literature I could find related to Chronic Fatigue Syndrome and coexisting conditions. I inundated my brain with information about medications, symptoms and treatments. I was driven to learn all that was out there to know. The amount of information available was abundant.

As I learned more, I began to wonder why there wasn't much media coverage about CFS. Years later, I still wonder why a light isn't shone on this debilitating illness when it impacts so many people. It sneaks up on people as a burglar sneaks into a house under the cover of darkness. It, then, violates the sufferer's life, stealing his/her vitality, memory, self-confidence, friends, employment, education and dreams. It leaves a path of destruction like a tornado through the wide-open plains. Health, families, relationships and plans are swiftly pulled from their foundations and thrown haphazardly in the rubble left behind. Why isn't the general-public aware this is out there?

For the first time in my life, I visited support chat rooms. I sought advice and information from adults who live with the disease. They were open and compassionate.

Their hearts went out to Anthony because of his youth. They literally walked me through the early stages of Anthony's illness.

On a message board, I sought ideas to encourage Anthony. Bobbi, the mother of an 18-year-old boy responded first. This was my confirmation that boys get it, too. Surprisingly, four children also responded. Two of them reached out to Anthony and formed friendships with him when he most needed to hear from others who understood exactly what he was going through. Via Instant Messaging, they talked, complained, laughed and teased.

Through the Internet, God blessed me with Becky, another mom, who I could ask questions and turn to in my frustrations. How comforting it was to have another parent who understood our plight. She led me to an Internet support group for parents of children with CFS. They embraced me and walked me through the first two years. At first, I felt sorely inadequate to provide support or encouragement to people who had been in the trenches longer than I.

The next pages focus on much of the information from my workshops. Please feel free to use this information to help every child with CFS you know.

Chapter Twelve:
Protecting Their Education from the CFS Hurricane

Three years ago, I developed a workshop focused on CFIDS and the impact on a child's education. The staff members who have attended include: school nurses, librarians, administrators, social workers, psychologists, guidance counselors, foreign language instructors, P.E. teachers, physical therapists, occupational therapists, vision specialists, assistive technology specialists, speech-language pathologists, special and general education teachers.

After the informative portion of the workshop, the educators are given the opportunity to immediately put what they've learned into action. They are broken into teams and encouraged to brainstorm over case studies of children with CFIDS. They have all been focused and deliberate in their task. They take this endeavor seriously and have helped many children. I applaud them for their efforts.

The information below is a compiled list of my ideas and suggestions and input from the dedicated educators who have participated in these workshops.

The student's disability affects his/her performance in the following areas:

- Written work (expression, spelling, speed, legibility, copying)
- Reading skills (decoding, comprehension)
- Math skills (computation, reasoning)
- Listening-comprehension skills

- Oral-expression skills
- Attention/concentration for extended time
- Gross and/or fine motor skills
- Peer and/or social behaviors
- Organizational skills
- Emotional/Behavioral

Setting

- Preferential Seating (easy access to door, near area of instruction or near the window for natural lighting)
- Small Group (prevents sensory overload)
- Homebound services (immune system dysfunction, pain, fatigue)
- Modified school day (full day, half day, homebound)
- This depends on the severity of the symptoms of the child.
- *Keep student's work area free of unnecessary materials.*

Assignments

- **Shortened assignments** (once a student has mastered a concept, move on)
- **Reduced pencil/paper tasks** (due to pain in small muscles and joints in hands)
- **Extended Time** (fluctuations in disease contradict time limitations)
- **Opportunity to respond orally** (when pain in hands is too severe. . . per request)

- Allow student to obtain and report information utilizing recorder, interviews and fact sheets.
- Allow student to begin projects early.
- Design assignments to be graded on specific parts of the writing process.
- Encourage student to use graph paper to organize math problems on paper.
- Alternative books or materials on same topic
- Videotapes in place of text
- Projects substituted for written reports (collages, videotaped when too ill to attend school)
- Use of graphic organizers
- Allow cursive or print (depending on ability of hands)
- Provide math worksheets with problems already written
- Break writing assignments into segments of shorter tasks

Instruction/Methods

- **Assignment Notebooks** (filled out and/or checked by teacher and parents daily)
- **Highlight key words on handouts, notes and study guides**
- **Peer Tutor/Helper** (to assists with disorientation problems)
- **Frequent/Immediate feedback** (necessary to be certain the student is on the right track)
- **Repetition of instruction**
- **Student responses on tape** (when manual response is too painful or fatigue too severe)

- **Additional directions** (clarify, repeat, reword)
- **Supplement with visual cues**
- **Minimize the usage of overhead projector** *(visual dysfunction)*
- **Reduce amount of copying from text, board and overheads**
- **Present assignments in sequential steps**
- **Avoid cluttered worksheets**
- **Use concrete examples of concepts before teaching abstract**
- **Reduce the number of concepts taught at one time.**
- **Supply written directions to supplement verbal cues.**
- **In science, provide lab sheets with highlighted instructions.**

Other

- **Tape record all lessons.** (assists in recall and processing deficits)
- **Recorder/Scribe** (daily notes provided)*scribe must copy exactly what the student says and allow the student to correct mistakes
- **Video recorded classes.**
- **Email assignments to home.**
- **Check on organization of student's notebook.**
- **Provide the opportunity for movement.** *(standing, squatting, kneeling, placing head on desk)*
- **Monitor frustration and tolerance levels.**
- **Allow for delayed processing time in student's responses.**

Materials/Technology

- **Taped Text Books/Materials** (visual dysfunction, short-term memory, comprehension)
- **Highlighted Text/Materials** (key points on handouts, notes and study guides)
- **Large Print/Magnification** (at least 14pt for visual dysfunction)
- **Calculator/Math charts** (dyscalculia)
- **Spell Check on assignments** (memory, sequencing)
- **Access to keyboard/word processor** (reduces pain and increases legibility)
- **Study guides**
- **Small notebook with pictures, names, highlighted school map, condition explanation, address and phone number for disorientation issues**
- **Overlays** *(break the glare from fluorescent lights and contrast of black print on white paper)*
- **Assignment Notebook**

Other

- **Course syllabus** *(provided so student has plenty of time to work on upcoming projects. Student can also take advantage of up time to get ahead of the down times)*
- **Provide ruler or index card** *(to keep place when reading)*

Behavior

- **Frequent Breaks** *(scheduled rest breaks to prevent "crashes")*
- **Quiet Time**

Testing Accommodations

Timing/Scheduling

- **Flexible schedule**
- **Extended time**
- **Breaks**
- **Multiple settings**

Setting

- **Group size: small groups, individual testing**
- **Natural lighting**

Environmental modifications

- **Lighting**
- **Adaptive furniture**
- **Location**
- **Preferential seating**
- **Hospital/home**

Presentation

- **Visual aids**
- **Magnifying glass**
- **Templates**
- **Masks or markers**
- **Test by sections not chapters**
- **Word banks**
- **Multiple choice**
- **Chunk like concepts**

Font

Large print test or increased size answer bubble

Directions

- **Assistance with directions reading, simplifying, repeating**
- **Tape recorder**
- **Audio taped version of test items**

Response

- **Mark in booklet**
- **Student responds verbally**

Math aids

- **Abacus**
- **Math tables**
- **Calculator**

Writing instruments

- **Large diameter or pencil grip**
- **Word Processor/Typewriter**
- **Any other assistive tech they use regularly for academic work**

Spelling aids

- **Spell checker**
- **Spelling dictionary**

Extra Suggestions For Needs Related To Cfids

- **Study carrel** *(minimize distractions)*
- **Second set of books for home** *(eliminates added pain and fatigue)*
- **Laminated hall pass**
- **Ice chips or cold water** *(temperature fluctuations)*
- **Wheelchair/Scooter at door**
- **Release from classes five minutes early.** *(minimizes sensory disturbances)*
- **Eye drops** *(dry, scratchy eyes)*
- **Jacket kept in class** *(temperature fluctuations)*

- **Elevator privileges**
- **Classrooms in same area**
- **Snack breaks when necessary** *(nausea, digestive disorders)*
- **Mints/ginger ale** *(nausea)*
- **Highlighted map** *(disorientation issues)*
- **PE modification, exemption or Physical therapy substituted for P.E.**
- **Change of clothing in nurse's office** *(abdominal issues)*
- **Allowed to have water at desk** *(throat and orthostatic intolerance issues)*
- **NO Cafeteria** *(sound, motion, odor sensitivities)*
- **Allow student to have lunch in a quiet area with a few friends.**
- **Dim lighting** *(allow use of sun glasses or brimmed hat)*
- **Minimize usage of overhead projector.**
- **Caution with sciences** *(chemical compounds)*, **cologne usage, cleaning products** *(chemical sensitivity)*
- **Laminated Nurse's Pass** *(unlimited usage)*
- **Referrals to Related Services** *(Occupational Therapist, Physical Therapist, Dietitian, Vision Therapist)*
- **Speech-Language Therapist or Assistive Tech** *(for evaluation.)*
- **Consider available community resources.**
- **Alert school nurse in reference to the student.**
- **Allow use of comfort measures.** *(ice pack, analgesic rub, heat patches)*

Homebound Needs

- Special-education teacher preferred.
- Instruction scheduled at best time of day *for child*
- Web cam in classroom to enable the student to have contact with others on a regular basis.

Physical Therapist

- Stretching
- Walking
- Manual Therapy
- Water Therapy
- Help student recognize when his/her body is reaching its limits.

School Counselor

- Help student learn relaxation techniques
- Help child establish ways to communicate specific levels of pain, cognitive delay, pain, dizziness, etc.
- Inform staff of the chosen methods.

School Nurse

- Ice chips and/or cold water *(temperature fluctuations)*
- Change of clothing *(digestive dysfunction)*
- Inform parent(s) when viruses, flu, etc are going

through school.
- **Keep emergency numbers handy**
- **Familiarize yourself with child's pain scales and establish with parents the appropriate level to call home.**
- **"Care Kit" in office containing**
  o **Crackers, ginger ale, mints** *(nausea)*
  o **Eye drops** *(dry eyes)*
  o **Hot/cold pack**
  o **Analgesic rub**

Assistive Technology

- **Computer software that focuses on writing process, memory, etc**
- **Speech-recognition Software**
- **Encourage the student to acquire keyboarding skills**
- **Mouse-driven computer programs**

Occupational Therapy

- **Positioning devices to support trunk, neck, arms, wrists**
- **Observe student in learning environment.**
- **Position materials and computer/keyboard to conserve energy**
- **Modified pencils, pens, art equipment**
- **Slant board**
- **Keyboarding skills**

Speech/language Pathologist

- **Strategies for reading comprehension**
- **Strategies for auditory comprehension and memory**
- **Attention process training**
- **Organizational Skills**
- **Strategies for delayed processing when fatigued and trying to verbalize in general conversation or in the educational setting**

Vision Specialist

- **Visual-Otopic screening** *(to determine correct color overlay for child)*
- **Possible referral to vision specialist and/or vision therapist**

P.E.

- **Once student is able to return to class, participation MUST be adapted to the child's specific needs and tolerance levels by specialist.**
- **Exemption from P.E. or substitution of physical therapy**
- **Modified P.E.**

Transportation

- **Be sure of what kind of transportation student requires** *(wheelchair lift, general, special* *education)*

- **Make sure child's bus drivers are informed about CFS**
- **Have a plan in place for bad weather days**
- **Have a plan in place for late openings, ½ days and early outs**

HAVE A CRISIS PLAN IN PLACE FOR THE WORST-CASE SCENARIO

EVERY STAFF MEMBER WHO COMES INTO CONTACT WITH THE CHILD MUST BE INFORMED ENTIRELY ABOUT THE CHILD'S DISEASE. THIS INCLUDES TEACHERS, NURSES, BUS DRIVERS, CUSTODIANS, PARA PROFESSIONALS, OFFICE STAFF AND ADMINISTRATORS. *(Because they look "fine", they are often overlooked until a crisis arises.)*

Chapter Thirteen:
My Suggestions

Educational

1. Document. Document! DOCUMENT!! Keep record of all meetings, phone conversations, written correspondence, messages and face-to-face interactions.

2. Educate yourself as much as you can about your child's disease and the symptoms that are specific to your child.

3. Provide the staff with the opportunity to become informed about the disease. *(pamphlets, brochures, workshops, web links, books, videos, etc)*

4. Keep communication open between you and the people who are responsible for your child's education.

5. Know that your input is as important as anyone's on the Child Study, Eligibility or IEP committee.

6. When possible and appropriate, allow your child to take part in the meetings.

7. Have notes ready before each meeting so you can stay focused on the issues that need to be addressed for your child.

8. Have someone who knows your child well go with you to meetings.

9. Learn all you can about your and your child's rights in the education process.

10. Stay aware about the implementation of your child's IEP. Once you've got it on paper, you need to make sure it's in effect. Your child's future will be affected one way or the other.

11. If you have questions, call to speak with the teacher, case manager or administrator before things get out of hand.

- I don't wear rose-colored glasses and my name is not Polyanna. I just wanted to give you a place to start. If these things get you nowhere, the IDEA provides a process for mediation and/or complaint.

Medical

1. Keep your own copies of all of your child's records.

2. Share information on research findings, medical journals and articles pertinent to your child's disease with the doctor.

3. Remember, nobody knows everything…not even doctors.

4. Don't be afraid to look elsewhere.

5. Remember that no matter what, you and your child are entitled to be treated with respect and dignity.

6. Don't be afraid to ask for a second opinion.

7. Remember that even though you may not have your PhD or MD, you do have your M.O.M or D.A.D.

8. Know the effects and side effects of each medication. *(many of our children are hyper sensitive to certain medications)*

Personal

1. Listen to how your child feels. Ask, then really listen.

2. Encourage your child to continue to look at his/her goals. Together, brainstorm about ways to achieve the goals by going around the disability.

3. Encourage some level of social interaction.

4. Reassure the child that your frustration is not his/her fault.

5. Find a source of support and encouragement for yourself.

6. Let the child know that you accept him/her as he/she is now (don't put so much emphasis on finding

a cause or cure that you neglect the blessing that is in front of you).

7. Never give up hope.

8. Have a plan. (example: This is how we're going to do this if you're not well by then) By doing this, they know there is a chance they might improve. They also know the disease won't completely stop them if they don't)

Miscellaneous

1. Share your experience with others.

2. Share your information with others.

3. Don't be afraid to ask for help from others who have been or are still where you are.

4. Set aside time to do what gives you pleasure.

5. Find humor in some of the symptoms *(sometimes, all we can do is laugh)*.

6. Don't forget the rest of the family.

7. See what community services may be available.

8. Always have a "plan B"

- Remember that God knows how strong you are even if you doubt it at times. He may have plans for you to become an advocate, volunteer, counselor or homebound teacher for these children.

Chapter Fourteen:
From A Mother's Heart

In the years since Anthony became ill, I've been forced to go to battle often. Many people just don't understand. This includes friends, family, educators, doctors, nurses and counselors. It is hard to feel like you always have to be on your guard. I've lost my husband, but my Heavenly Father immediately stepped in and walked me through. The Lord Himself goes before you and will be with you; He *will never leave you nor forsake you. Do not be afraid; do not be discouraged. ~ Deuteronomy 31:8*

This is not a story of woe. This is a story of hope. My son has not recovered. I don't know that I'll ever have the same son I had before, but I praise God for the one I have. He knows the plans he has for us each and every one!

For those of you who are fighting this battle, please hold on and know that you're not alone. There are people out here who care and will try to help you learn to live life in spite of this cooperative disease. You just have to keep fighting. If we stop, what happens to the people who come after us? Someone has to keep up the fight. I pray that an Aaron or a Becky touches your lives.

I sometimes get asked what my advice is to people who come into contact with people who have CFS. Believe the person. Be patient with the person. Understand that the disease is on its own schedule, and figure out a time when you can adjust your schedule so you can spend some peak time with that person. Read to them. Talk to them about your life so they can keep up with life outside of the house. Don't compare his or her symptoms and/or rate of recovery with someone else's. Offer to take them and go with them to appointments. Learn about the disease. Make them laugh (sometimes this requires acting quite foolish, but their laughter is worth millions!) Accept the person in front of you as that person is right now. If they could return to their old selves, they would. If they're depressed, encourage them to seek a counselor. *****SCREEN THE COUNSELOR WELL, FIRST. If the counselor doesn't believe this disease is a real physical disease... keep looking. If they've never heard of the disease...keep looking. If they're not willing to learn about the disease... keep looking.

As I write this book, there is no cure all out there for this disease. There are only theories about where it came from and what causes it. There are several groups looking for answers. Be careful what methods of treatment you try. You don't want anything that will make the condition worse.

In the time that's passed since Anthony first became ill with his digestive problems, I have learned a lot. People have jokingly told me than I need to go for my medical degree or write a book. I chose the latter.

My prayer is that the manner in which we sail on this journey will bring glory to our Father in Heaven. I pray that whatever I say is expressed with dignity and restraint when I'm called to stand strong in conflict over my son. My prayer is that the battle become a bit easier for the next person because of the steps we have taken and the progress we have made. I pray that many people will read this and at least develop empathy for those around them who fall ill with this, or any other, disease.

Do I hold a grudge against the people who seemed to have been stumbling blocks in our path? I don't have the time or energy to waste on holding a grudge. I know that in the future, I will not allow doctors, educators, counselors, etc., so much time while I hope for a change in their attitude. I do pray that they increase their knowledge enough about the disease they won't treat the next person that comes their way with CFS in the same manner. If they aren't willing to learn, I pray that God keeps people with CFS from being exposed to them. In retrospect, I have come to appreciate the challenges that have been placed into our path, because they have revealed the strength we've developed in Christ. Would we be as bold? Would our bond be so close? I praise God for His plan, and am honored to travel it with His light as our beacon.

I have learned that we all bring with us different cultural views, personalities, opinions and life experiences. There are nurses, educators, adults with CFS, home schooling parents, etc. These differences end up being beneficial. We must all apply our own unique gifts, talents and knowledge bases to each other's circumstances. It's so much easier to think outside of the box when we have no emotions involved.

Once I realized that I was capable of helping other parents travel this journey, I established a web site putting my favorite resources together for parents and educators. My hope was to make research less tedious and more easily accessible. I hoped this would encourage educators to learn more while forming a bridge between the educators and the parents.

I also started a support group for people of all ages with Chronic Fatigue Syndrome and Fibromyalgia. We have shared a treasure of information, encouragement and feelings.

Finally, I had to approach the arena in which I faced the most conflict. I had to decide if I wanted to make a difference for other children and parents or just be satisfied by taking care of my own. *Praise be to God and the Father of our Lord Jesus Christ, the Father of compassion and the God of all comfort who comforts us in all our troubles, so that we can comfort those in any trouble with the comfort we ourselves have received from God. ~ 2 Corinthians 1:3,4*

From that verse, my decision was made. I decided to use what I had learned from working in Special Education to help, first Anthony. Once I started to figure out techniques, accommodations and modifications that were helpful to him, I created a presentation for educators. The first one was given for Anthony's school system and it was a success. All of the evaluations were positive.

I then started going to select schools in other states, when asked. I noted the success and awareness continued, so I continue to speak whenever I can.

My next goal was to publish this book to reach as many parents and school systems as possible. I want to prevent children, parents and educators from experiencing the negative journey we had to travel.

Know this, all who read this. I am NOTHING without Jesus Christ. I would not be so bold, if God haven't given me such a wonderful son for whom I couldn't help but fight. I couldn't speak in front of others if God didn't give me the strength and courage to do so. Parents, hang on to your faith! Love your children. Stand up for your children, because nobody else *(not doctors, teachers, insurance companies, etc)* will stand beside your child reaping the benefits or suffering the consequences of the decisions that are made today.

One internal struggle I face is the fact that I've raised my son to respect all adults. On top of that, he doesn't like attention on himself. With this disease, those characteristics place a child in a Catch-22 situation. I was also raised believing teachers and doctors were experts and authorities. I have had to pray about these things and then talk with Anthony about the answers I have come up with. No man is a god *(all-knowing and all-seeing)*. We respect that these people have gone through schools to occupy positions they hold. On the other hand, we have to acknowledge that they don't know everything. Sometimes we have to advocate and self-advocate for things we know are right. Feelings might get hurt, but we cannot allow that to deter us from the path we must follow. We might never be capable of changing their minds, but we must try. We must take up the battle where the ones who came before us left off. Fight the good fight for our selves and the ones who will follow us. If someone acknowledges our effort on the journey, that's a blessing. If we never get recognized, we await the day that Jesus tells us face-to-face that we have "fought the good fight…that our race has been won.

Welcome home faithful servant…well done!"

Chapter Fifteen:
Witness on a Stormy Sea

Most times, when people, who knew us before, see Anthony in his wheelchair, they are filled with a mixture of emotion. Some cry. Some don't know how to respond. Some want him to have a miraculous healing. Some want to baby him. Most people want to feel sorry for Anthony. I will not allow it.

If Anthony falls, he still gets back up. Even if he needs help, he gets back up. Anthony uses a wheelchair, but that chair is his FREEDOM! Anthony can't do all he used to do…but Anthony is doing much more than he was able to do three years ago. Anthony is quiet. My son is a listener.

For the people who question God's decision of giving my son this cross to bear, we need to remember that God knows and sees all. If not, a bird falls from the sky without Him knowing, He knows that Anthony is down here suffering. There is a purpose in everything He allows people to endure. He NEVER has left Anthony's side. He gives Anthony the tools that he needs to endure this trial.

In the weakness of this journey, I have seen Anthony develop a quiet strength and wisdom beyond his years. He is full of compassion. He is an advocate for those who cannot advocate for themselves. He has an insight that he could never get from a textbook.

For the first time since he became ill, we were actually able to travel this summer. We traveled to Georgia to visit Janet, Jerry and Dani. Anthony enjoyed Janet's grandchildren while teasing Dani as if they were brother and sister. We traveled to Florida to see Jay and Dina. We attended a family reunion. Anthony was actually able to travel with me to a workshop in Illinois where we stayed with Linda and Megan. It's been a long time and we appreciate the blessing of the travel God allowed us.

Anthony recognizes how easy it is to take for granted the simple things in life. He knows it's easy to praise God and rejoice in the gifts He gives when life sails by on crystal-clear waters. He also knows that his testimony is even stronger by the example he sets by leaning on God even more when life throws storms in his path.

This is the biggest trial we've ever faced together. We've held on to each other and we have held on to Christ. We also have held on to his dreams. He still wants to be a medical-research scientist. If it's in my power, I'll find a way for him to realize that dream because that's my job. *That is why, for Christ's sake, I delight in weakness, in* insults, in hardships, in persecutions, in difficulties. For when I am weak, then I am strong. ~2 Corinthians 12:10

Resources

These resources have supplied us with much needed guidance.

- A Doctor's Guide to CFS Dr. David S. Bell
- A Parent's Guide to CFS Dr. David S. Bell, Mary Z. Robinson
- Faces of CFS Dr. David S. Bell
- M.E. The New Plague Jane Colby
- The Fainting Phenomenon Dr. Blair Grubb, Mary McMann
- Fibromyalgia & Chronic Myofascial Pain Syndrome Dr. Devin Starlanyl
- Coping with Your Child's Chronic Illness Alesia T. Singer
- Vision and School Success George D. Spache, Ph.D., Lillian R. Hinds, Ph. D., Lois B. Bing, A.B., O.D.
- *Young People w/ Chronic Fatigue Syndrome Parent/Teacher Bridge Builder* http://groups.msn.com/YPWCParentTeacherBridgeBuilder
- *Pediatric Network (CFS/FM/OI)* www.pediatricnetwork.org
- *CFIDS Association of America* www.cfids.org
- *National CFIDS Foundation* www.ncf-net.org
- *National Fibromyalgia Association* www.fmaware.org
- *National Dysautonomia Research Foundation* www.ndrf.org
- *Recordings for the Blind and Dyslexic* www.rbfd.org

- *P.A.V.E. Parents Advocating for Vision Education* www.pave-eye.com
- *Children's Vision Information Network* www.childrenvision.com/studies_and_research.htm
- *Ehler's Danlos National Foundation EDNF-KIDS* www.ednf.org/children.php

About the Author

Shanon McQuown has worked as a paraprofessional in Special Education for several years. She has had the honor of working with children with Mild and Moderate Mental Disabilities, Traumatic Brain Injury, Autism, Learning Disabilities, and Emotional Disturbance. She lives in Northern Virginia with her parents and her son, the inspiration for this book, Anthony.

Since Anthony became ill, Shanon has trained as a Special Education Coach through the Parent Educational Advocacy Training Center (PEATC). She was a member of Partners in Policymaking (an organization that trains people to advocate for people with disabilities). Shanon has been a member of her county's Special Education Advisory Committee (SEAC) for the past two years.

Shanon firmly believes that disabilities place limits on people's lives…but the disability is not THE limit. Her desire is to spare other children from having to journey on the same rough voyage Anthony traveled by raising awareness across the nation. By doing this, the struggles will not seem as if they were in vain.

www.ingramcontent.com/pod-product-compliance
Lightning Source LLC
Chambersburg PA
CBHW020418290526
45785CB00002B/614